ear candling

in essence

Mary Dalgleish and Lesley Hart

Series Editor: Nicola Jenkins

Hodder Arnold

A MEMBER OF THE HODDER HEADLINE GROUP

Orders: please contact Bookpoint Ltd, 130 Milton Park, Abingdon, Oxon OX14 4SB. Telephone: (44) 01235 827720. Fax: (44) 01235 400454. Lines are open from 9.00 – 5.00, Monday to Saturday, with a 24 hour message answering service. You can also order through our website **www.hoddereducation.co.uk**

If you have any comments to make about this, or any of our other titles, please send them to
educationenquiries@hodder.co.uk

British Library Cataloguing in Publication Data
A catalogue record for this title is available from the British Library

ISBN-10: 0 340 92694 5
ISBN-13: 978 0 340 926 949

First Edition Published 2006
Impression number   10 9 8 7 6 5 4 3 2
Year   2009 2008 2007 2006

Hodder Headline's policy is to use papers that are natural, renewable and recyclable products and made from wood grown in sustainable forests. The logging and manufacturing processes are expected to conform to the environmental regulations of the country of origin.

Cover photo by Carl Drury
Artwork by Oxford Designers and Illustrators
Typeset by Servis Filmsetting Ltd, Manchester
Printed in Great Britain for Hodder Arnold, an imprint of Hodder Education, a member of the Hodder Headline Group, 338 Euston Road, London NW1 3BH by CPI Bath

acknowledgements

We would like to express our heartfelt thanks to the following people for their support in writing this manuscript:

Tamsin Smith at Hodder, who made it possible for us to write a book on this fascinating topic, and Nicola Jenkins who encouraged us to be a part of the series; Claire Baranowski and everyone at Hodder who was involved in creating this beautiful book; Jacquie Hawkins, Kate Harris, Linda Ayers, and Annette Tierney who reviewed our proposal, and made helpful suggestions; Biosun who provided images and research data and Kerry Curtis at Revital for facilitating this for us; Robert Eames, UK distributor for Otosan ear cones for information and pictures; Eva McNamara, Janice Micallef and Anne-Marie Cogdell for their valued help with research, and Caroline Bray who started us on our ear candling journey; our friends, colleagues, students and practitioners who sent in stories of their success with ear candling (Gabriele Steen, Luma Zaki, Penny Airs, Gurjit Panesar, Linda Gilham, Rosi Maldonado France, Lucretia Bertram-Smith, Linda Ayers). Particular thanks are also owed to our families, especially Patrick Doyle for all his help and patience with computer issues! For us, it has been a wonderful learning process and we hope it can inspire you to enjoy this ancient and wonderful therapy safely and effectively.

The author and publishers would like to thank the following for the use of photographs in this volume:

p3 (left) © Tom Bean/Corbis, p3 (top right) p15, p16 (left), p64 Courtesy of Biosun, p3 (bottom right) Photodisc, p4 Jen Smith Photography/Photographers Direct, p8 and p9 (left) Nigel Cattlin/Holt/FLPA, p9 (right) Bob Gibbons/Holt/FLPA, p10 TopFoto/Image Works, p11 (left) Science Photo Library (right) Nigel Cattlin/Holt/FLPA, p12 and p46 Rosie Mayer/Holt/FLPA, p13 Jean Hall/Holt/FLPA, p14 © Sergio Pitamitz/Zefa/Corbis, p16 (right) Courtesy of Malozza Distribution Ltd, p17 Kari Erik Marttila Photography/Photographers Direct, p20 (top), p23 Tracy Hebden/quaysidegraphics.com/Photographers Direct (bottom) Bo Viesland, MI&I/SPL, p20 Photodisc, p26 (left) Courtesy www.healer.ch, p36 Micromedics, p52 © Eliseo Fernandez/Reuters/Corbis, p53 and p56 Dr P Marazzi/SPL, p54 © Darama/Corbis, p63 © Mindak Art/Photographers Direct, p69 AJ Photo/SPL, p95 Marja Airio/Rex Features

Commissioned photographs by Carl Drury.

With thanks to our model, Anthea Scott.

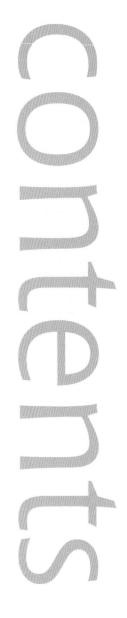

introduction

In today's materialistic, externally focused culture, it is easy to lose the belief that we can influence our own health; instead we rely on an external agent, a doctor or a pill in most cases, to fix us when we are ill. Yet study after study, as well as many personal histories published in health magazines and newspapers, show that people who take an active role in their own healthcare tend to have more positive results than those who do not. Many of us are waking up to the fact that we really can do a lot to maintain our health and wellbeing, and we are looking to complementary therapies to empower us on our journey. It is estimated that around 5.75 million people a year in the UK visit a complementary practitioner for treatment.

This growing awareness has been noticed by the government, and as far back as November 2000, a House of Lords Select Committee reported that 'the use of complementary and alternative medicine (CAM) is widespread and increasing across the developed world.' (See Bibliography for full details of this report.)

Even though they are frequently grouped together in one category, a distinction may be made between *complementary* and *alternative* medicine. Complementary therapies do not focus on diagnosing or curing a disease but can be used simultaneously with conventional medicine, to reduce side effects and stress and to increase wellbeing. Alternative therapies such as osteopathy, chiropractic, acupuncture, herbal medicine and homeopathy have an individual diagnostic approach and can in some instances be used in place of conventional medicine.

The Select Committee proposed three groups of CAM therapies, with the above five disciplines regarded as the 'most organised' professions, and making up the first group. Osteopathy and chiropractic are regulated by law while the others are at various stages of regulation. The second group contains bodywork therapies, which do not embrace diagnostic skills and are most often used to complement conventional medicine. The third group includes therapies which offer diagnostic information as well as treatment, but 'in general favour a philosophical approach and are indifferent to the scientific principles of conventional medicine', according to the report. The report also stressed the issues of public health policy raised by this growth, and recommended research, adequate information and sound practitioner training to ensure the safety of treatments available to the public.

With these same aims in mind, the Prince of Wales's Foundation for Integrated Health published 'Complementary Healthcare, a Guide for Patients' in February 2005. The aim of this guide is to help members of the public make informed choices about complementary therapies, and to find properly trained and qualified practitioners. The Prince of Wales's Foundation for Integrated Health (originally named the Foundation for Integrated Medicine) was formed in 1993 at the personal initiative of His Royal Highness The Prince of Wales, who is now its president. It aims to facilitate the development of safe, effective and efficient forms of healthcare to patients and their families, by supporting the development and delivery of integrated healthcare. This means encouraging conventional and complementary practitioners to work together to integrate their approaches.

The Foundation acts as a forum to promote and support discussion, and as centre for driving forward the integrated healthcare agenda. Separate professional organisations within individual disciplines are realising the need for common standards and research studies on the effectiveness of their treatments, in order to be taken more seriously; eg the Reflexology Forum, which incorporates various reflexology organisations.

Looking to the past, we can see that our ancestors left an incredible legacy of healing knowledge, and many of their practices have been rediscovered for use in the modern world. The ancient art of ear candling is one such healing tool, and our aim in writing this book is to present this rediscovered art for complementary practitioners wishing to include this therapy safely and effectively in their practice, as well as for the interest of the general public. For those wishing to practise professionally, there are details of accredited courses at the end of the book.

An ear candling treatment requires a pair of specialised 'candles' to be used in the ears; these 'candles' are in fact hollow tubes made from linen, cotton or hemp and hardened with beeswax which has been infused with honey and various herbs. The burning of these candles has many therapeutic effects, and a practitioner usually follows this with a gentle massage of the face, ears, neck and scalp to enhance the effects of the 'candling'.

It is a pleasant and non-invasive treatment that can be used to promote an enhanced state of health, to relieve conditions related to the ear and head area, or simply as an enjoyable means of relieving stress. In our modern age, conditions such as headaches and sinus problems are extremely common and can affect sufferers on a daily basis. Relief from such problems is very much in demand, and there is a growing trend to seek more natural forms of treatment.

Ear candling is commonly known as Hopi ear candling, acknowledging the fact that it was the Hopi Indians of the USA who kept this ancient practice alive and reintroduced it to the modern world. Other names given to ear candling include thermal-auricular therapy, funnelling, coning and other names which have been trademarked. The demand for this treatment has increased dramatically over the last 10–20 years and is being performed by many complementary health practitioners. In our practice we have seen a huge increase in ear candling, a growing demand for treatments and training courses (including students working within the NHS), and a curiosity as to what this fascinating therapy can do.

history

Our ancestors lived in small groups and tribes, close to nature. Survival meant connecting to the elements and understanding the use of nature. Humans sought understanding and knowledge of healing using a variety of tools. In many traditions, there is no distinction between medicine and religion; the Shaman or Medicine Man cares for mind, body and spirit.

Before organised religions, shamanic cultures existed around the world, and these cultures left behind a wealth of healing knowledge. Shamanism can be dated back over 50,000 years to the Stone Age people, and is the oldest form of human effort to connect with creation. The word 'shaman' comes from the language of an ancient tribe of reindeer herders in Siberia, and according to the *Encyclopaedia Britannica* it derives from the verb 'sa', which means 'to know'. Western anthropologists now apply the term 'shaman' to indigenous healers, visionaries and seers, and shamanic cultures still exist all over the world today, passing on their knowledge of healing to the wider community.

It is known that ear candling was practised by many ancient civilisations including the Aztecs, Greeks, Romans and Aborigines. The ancient Egyptians used reeds from the Nile coated with wax, packing mud around the ears to form a seal. Hollow twigs or cones made from glazed clay were also used to carry herbs or incense into the ears. It is generally accepted that the ear candling procedure was used not only for cleansing the ear canal but also for spiritual purification before initiation rites and rituals.

Ear candling was also widely practised in Italy, Spain, Romania and Asia, using materials such as rolled tobacco leaves and waxed cloth or paper, and these methods are still in use in some places.

According to old shamanic custom, traditional knowledge such as the ear candling procedure was passed on in oral form and through paintings. Historical pictorial records clearly show the use of ear candles in cultures across the globe. The most famous painting of the ear candling procedure is shown on an ancient rock painting in the Grand Canyon, USA.

Traditional practices faded out in many parts of the world, but in America some members of the native Hopi Indians kept the ear candling tradition alive. The Hopi are a Native American tribe who live primarily on a 1.5 million-acre reservation in north-eastern

casestudy

Eva, who was brought up in Spain and now lives in London, recalls ear candling as a regular part of her family routine:

'As a child, I loved swimming and spent a lot of time in the water. I often suffered from earaches and my mother or grandmother would make cones from paper infused with olive oil which they used to soothe my ears. It was a common practice where I lived.

I loved to lie down and feel the warmth of the smoke, and afterwards my mother would put a little piece of cotton wool in my ear and tell me to sleep on the side with my sore ear next to the pillow to keep it warm. My grandmother learned this technique from her mother, and she taught my mother who then taught me. In Spain, we use a special type of stiff paper which is used to wrap food in the grocery store. This paper absorbs the oil well and doesn't burn too quickly, although the flame can be quite big. My husband had chronic ear problems and was having his ears syringed at least twice a year as the wax kept building up and causing pain and deafness. It took me quite a while to convince him to allow me to use ear candles to help him. He thought it was some sort of witchcraft! He finally allowed me to try as he could see that syringing was only making the problem worse, stripping away all the wax and leaving the ear more vulnerable to infection. It also appeared to result in the production of excessive earwax, just as using cotton buds to clean the ears frequently seems to do. He has been having regular treatments for over a year now and has not needed to visit the doctor in that time. I still make my own ear cones with the paper which my mother sends me from Spain, but I would not advise anyone else to do this unless you know exactly what you are doing, as the ear is a very delicate organ.'

Arizona. They are renowned for their extensive knowledge of healing and their spiritual lifestyle, and more than most Native American peoples, they continue to practise some aspects of their traditional ceremonial culture. The translation of the word 'Hopi' means 'peaceful ones', and within this tribe there were various clans, each with differing practices. Although the Hopi did not call them 'ear candles', the Hopi Fire Clan used rolled waxed leaves infused with herbs as part of their spiritual ceremonies. The Hopi candles used today are named after this tribe

who first introduced this gentle therapy to the West (with the professional involvement of a German company called Biosun). The ear candles have evolved from the use of *fire*, *heat*, *smoke* and *herbs*, which all have healing qualities in their own right.

Fire has fascinated mankind throughout history, and this element has been used to give light and warmth, cook food and accompany religious ceremonies and rituals. Fire is considered to be a cleansing element in many cultures. Shamans believe that fire releases that part of yourself which no longer serves

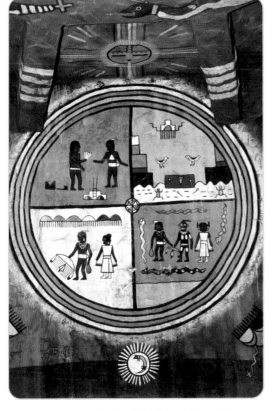

Coloured wall mural in the Hopi Tower, Grand Canyon

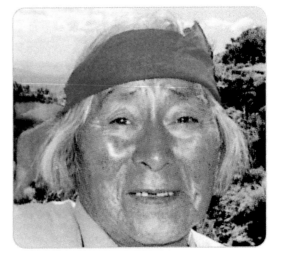

Martin Gashweseoma, traditional Hopi Elder and Guardian of the sacred stone tablets of the Hopi Clan

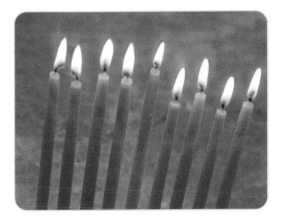

The fascination of fire

you. Fire is considered to clear negative energy on a spiritual and physical level. The ancients used fire extensively to promote healing; this could be a real fire or a simple candle.

Heat and cold were recognised by the ancients as a natural remedy for treating many bodily ailments. They discovered that heat is useful to relieve painful conditions such as aching muscles and earache, and that cold is useful to relieve inflamed conditions that follow injury. These natural healing methods are still widely used today. Scientifically, the application of heat stimulates the circulation and thus aids the healing process. Earaches due to infection are common among children,

and the practice of placing heat over the ear, perhaps in the form of a hot water bottle, is still appropriate in the modern age.

Smoke in a scented form was used in medieval Europe to drive out 'evil spirits', most likely using the herb *Hypericum perforatum* (St John's wort). This herb is used today in the treatment of depression.

Scented smoke is used in the ancient shamanic practice of burning bundles of aromatic herbs, known as smudge sticks; this traditional practice is still in use today. Negative energy is cleared from a space by wafting smouldering smudge sticks, perhaps in an area where there has been great unhappiness or sickness. This method known as 'smudging' is also used to facilitate healing on a physical level – by wafting the smoke around a person's aura or by blowing smoke into a person's ears. Sage is one of the primary herbs used, due to its cleansing and purifying properties.

Smudging is an alternative term for burning incense. Incense to produce scented smoke has been used in cultures all over the world since before recorded time, and is widely used today in major religions across the world. Burning incense during ceremonies stills a busy mind and brings people to enter a state of quietness and one more receptive to a higher level of consciousness.

Scientifically, burning herbs has been shown to promote negative ions (which make you feel well and energised, such as those near a waterfall), and diminish positive ions (which leave you feeling sluggish, such as those found near electric pylons).

In conclusion, ear candling has evolved as a user-friendly way of bringing together the well-known healing elements of fire, heat, burning candles and scented smoke, to a practice with a more tangible connection to the physical body.

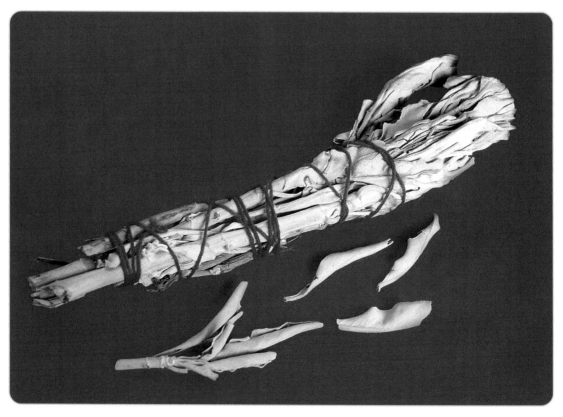

Sage smudge sticks

FAQs

Was one particular culture responsible for introducing ear candling in the ancient world?

Ear candling evolved independently in many cultures across the globe, at a time when these cultures had no means of communication. Man looked to nature for healing tools, and the use of ear candles in various forms would have been a natural progression from the use of healing elements such as fire, heat, burning candles and scented smoke.

I have heard of 'ear coning'; what does this mean?

In ancient times, this process was known as 'coning' because cone-shaped instruments made from glazed pottery clay were used. The shape of these created a downward spiral of the smoke and heated air, which carried the burning herbs to cleanse the ear canal. It also created a slight suction action to loosen debris, which may be in the ear canal. Some Indian tribes blow herbal smoke into the ear canal through a cone-shaped object, often rolled up paper. Some modern ear candles are cone-shaped.

Why are such instruments not in use today?

Due to health regulations, we now have to use disposable cones or funnel-shaped ear candles which have been rigorously tested to ensure safety during the process. For insurance purposes, products used by practitioners on their clients should conform to European regulations. Suppliers of such products are listed at the back of this book.

what are ear candles?

Ear candles are natural products. The term 'candle' is a bit of a misnomer since they are not candles as we usually understand them: they are hollow, have no wick and are usually made from cotton, cotton-flax or hemp fibres. Good quality ear candles are sourced from unbleached organically grown crops. The fibres are stiffened when they are sprayed with pure beeswax, and the basic ear candle is a simple as that. Many varieties include the addition of herbs and other ingredients with various therapeutic benefits.

Ear candling has received some negative publicity in recent years, with reports on various internet sites of injuries such as burns of the pinna and external auditory canal, partial or complete occlusion of the ear canal with candle wax, and tympanic membrane (eardrum) perforation. These accidents are usually due to the use of poor quality ear candles with no safety features, and lack of knowledge on the part of the person carrying out the treatment. The importation and sale of ear candles is currently prohibited in Canada, and no medical device licences have been approved for these products. All of this has led sceptics to claim that they are dangerous and have no effect, but on the other hand, there are many thousands of users who report excellent results and health benefits from their use.

Rather than decreasing in popularity, demand for ear candles has increased sharply in the USA, Middle East, UK and the rest of Europe. Now, there are several brands of ear candles and cones available, which have been rigorously tested for quality and safety, compliant with EU regulation 93/42/EEC and registered as a medical device in the EU. Following a training course in ear candling and the use of such products, a therapist can now feel confident in practising the art of ear candling.

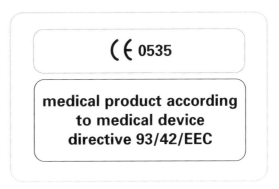

$C\epsilon$ 0535

medical product according to medical device directive 93/42/EEC

EU safety label

7

Constituents

The constituents of ear candles vary depending on the brand. Traditionally, ingredients such as chamomile, sage and honey were chosen for their benefits to the ear, nose and throat area, and their ability to stimulate the immune system. Many of the constituents including beeswax, chamomile, honey, propolis and sage are used today in the treatment of hay fever. Outlined below are examples of the constituents most commonly used in ear candle production today.

Cotton

Cotton is a soft fibre that grows around the seeds of the cotton plant. The fibre is spun into thread and used to make a soft,

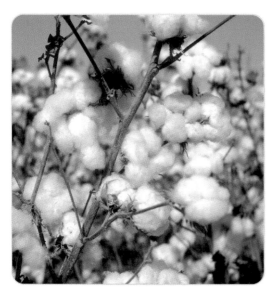

Cotton plant

breathable textile. Cotton is produced in many parts of the world, and the industry relies heavily on fertilisers and insecticides. The end product is often bleached to meet commercial requirements regarding colour. Good quality ear candles use organically grown unbleached cotton, often mixed with flax (linen) to produce a fabric which is soft and flexible. Most brands of candles are made from cotton flax, which burns cleanly without giving off any noxious fumes.

Linen (flax)

Linen is a vegetable fibre obtained from the inside of the woody stalk of the flax plant, which has a yellowish stem and bright blue flowers. The flax plant also supplies seeds (linseeds), which can be ground into flour for bread as well as crushed for oil and animal feed. Linseed oil is also an ingredient in many fine oil paints, varnishes and stains, and was used in the manufacture of linoleum. The use of linen, or 'flaxen cloth', dates back to people who lived about 10,000 years ago. These people dressed in animal skins but made coarse cloth and fish nets from flax. Fragments of the cloth and nets have been found in parts of Switzerland, the home of the Neolithic lake dwellers. Fine linens were used as the burial shrouds of the Egyptian Pharaohs, and Egyptian burial chambers depict flax cultivation and clothing made from flax fibres. Some ear candles are made from a mixture of cotton and linen, often referred to as cotton-flax.

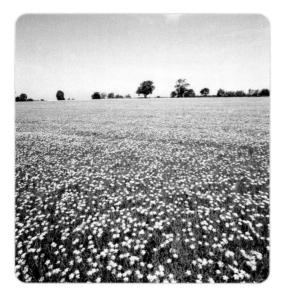

Linen plant

The seeds are an excellent nutritional source that can provide quality fats and proteins. Hemp seed oil is used for its healing qualities in many creams, ointments and cosmetics, but can also be used to create paint, varnishes and lubricants. The high fibre content of hemp makes it a natural resource for building materials, papermaking, and even biodegradable plastics. Hemp is a viable environmentally-sound energy source, which burns cleanly without producing noxious fumes.

Hemp

Some candles are made from hemp rather than cotton. Hemp is harvested for its fibres for hemp clothing and seeds for hemp oil. With a relatively short growth cycle of 100–120 days, it is an efficient and economical crop for farmers to grow. Due to the similar leaf shape, hemp is frequently confused with marijuana. Although both plants are from the plant species 'cannabis sativa', hemp contains virtually none of the active ingredient found in marijuana and has no illicit uses. The most commonly seen modern hemp product is clothing. Hemp clothing is warmer, softer, more absorbent and breathable, and significantly longer-lasting than clothing made from cotton.

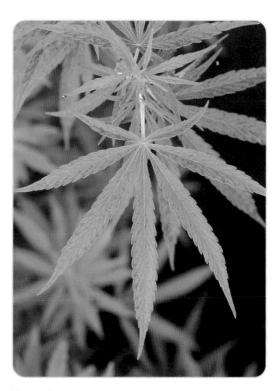

Hemp plant

Beeswax

Beeswax is made by worker bees, who use it to build comb cells in which the young are raised and honey and pollen are stored. The wax is made from a substance produced by glands on the surface of the bee's abdomen, which it mixes with pollen and propolis. Its colour varies from almost white to almost black, depending on the floral sources of the pollen and propolis. The young are raised in the brood comb area of the hive, and the wax from this area tends to be darker than the wax from the honeycomb as impurities accumulate more quickly in the brood comb.

The best quality beeswax is from the 'cappings' of the honeycomb – the part of the comb that seals in the honey collected by the bees. Cappings are sliced off the comb before the honey is harvested and these are sold to wax buyers for use in crafts and industry. About one to two pounds of wax is produced for every hundred pounds of honey.

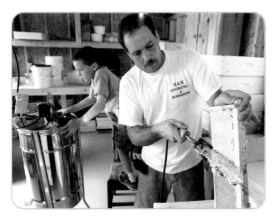

Removing beeswax cappings from a honeycomb

Beeswax is widely used in pharmaceutical and skincare products. It is antiseptic, anti-inflammatory and fights infections. For ear candles, beeswax is melted and infused with various ingredients such as herbs. The fabric (cotton, cotton-flax or hemp) which forms the basis of the ear candle is sprayed with or dipped into this mixture, which gives it shape and rigidity when it dries. Beeswax has hydrating qualities that help to soften and loosen compacted earwax.

Beeswax candles are widely used in places of worship as beeswax is non-toxic, burns cleanly with little or no wax dripping, and produces little visible smoke. This also makes it an ideal choice for therapeutic use in ear candles. It has an almost indefinite shelf life, and beeswax found in ancient Egyptian tombs has retained its pliability even after thousands of years.

Beta-carotene (Vitamin A)

Beta-carotene is the molecule that gives carrots their orange colour. It is part of a family of chemicals called carotenoids, which are found in many fruits and vegetables (particularly carrots), as well as some animal products such as egg yolks. Carotenoids were first isolated in the early nineteenth century and have been used as food colourings since the 1950s. Beta-carotene is most important as the precursor of vitamin A, and it also has antioxidant properties that may help in preventing disease. Its most significant benefit to ear candling is its ability to strengthen the immune system.

Chamomile

This is a perennial herb with small daisy-like flowers. The name 'chamomile' comes from Ancient Greek meaning 'earth apple', probably as it has a scent similar to apples. There are many types of chamomile – the one most commonly used in ear candles is roman chamomile (*Anthemis nobilis*). Chamomile has many medicinal properties, the most important being analgesic, anti-inflammatory, soothing and calming.

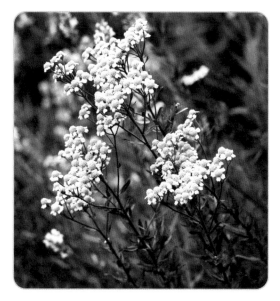

Roman chamomile (*Anthemis nobilis*)

On a physical level, it soothes inflamed skin and is used in the treatment of sunburn. It is helpful for painful conditions such as earache, headaches and sore throats. Chamomile is beneficial in allergic conditions and is often added to cosmetics as an anti-allergy agent. It is an immune stimulant and wards off infection. On an emotional level it relieves nervous tension and stress-related conditions, and aids restful sleep. Its actions are effective yet gentle, making it a good choice for treating both children and adults.

Honey

Honey is the sweet fluid produced by bees from flower nectar. After collecting the nectar and storing it in their stomachs (where some processing takes place), bees regurgitate it as sweet syrup (honey) and store it in their hive to provide them with food through the winter. Honey does not spoil because it has a high sugar concentration that kills bacteria, making it a natural preservative.

The healing properties of honey have been known for many centuries. Greek scholars such as Hippocrates and Aristotle used honey as a medicinal remedy for conditions such as skin disorders, sores and respiratory complaints. It has been used throughout the ages in the treatment of wounds – a common practice in the First World War. Cleopatra used honey to prevent wrinkling and to soften the skin. Honey is full of vitamins and

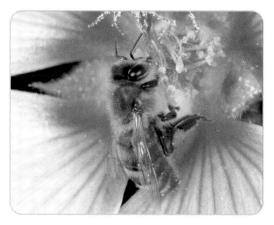

The honey bee provides many useful products

minerals and is at home both in the kitchen cupboard and the medicine chest. Its antiseptic qualities fight infection and it is used to soothe coughs and sore throats. It is a popular choice in skincare products due to its moisturising and hydrating qualities. Its hydrating qualities can help to soften and loosen compacted earwax.

Propolis

Propolis is a glue-like substance produced and used by bees to build and protect the hive. It is formed from resins collected by the bees from buds of poplar, birch and pine trees. They chew the resin, which mixes with their saliva to form propolis; they then use this to seal open spaces in the hive and to maintain hive hygiene, protecting themselves from disease.

Science has only recently recognised the importance of propolis, though its use goes back to Egyptian medical texts dating from 1550 BC. Hippocrates, the founder of modern medicine, recommended propolis to treat wounds, and the Roman naturalist Pliny claimed it could heal sores, reduce swellings and extract poison and pus from abscesses. It was used in folk medicine throughout the Middle Ages and listed as an official drug in the *London Pharmacopoeia*, a book published in 1618 for all London apothecaries (chemists or pharmacists), standardising remedies and listing the crude drugs used to make them. It was a traditional remedy for severe infections including malaria, tuberculosis and oral thrush. Nowadays it is widely available from health food stores in liquid form, capsules, tablets and ointments, and is an ingredient in Otosan ear cones and ear drops.

Sage

There are many varieties of sage; the one most commonly used in ear candles is *Salvia officinalis*. The name for this plant denotes its importance throughout history as a healing tool. Its Latin name *salvia* means salvation – this could either be salvation from physical illness or salvation on a spiritual level. The Roman name for sage, *herba sacra*, meaning sacred herb, indicates how much it was valued, and the Romans practised a special ceremony just to pick sage. Native American Indians traditionally used 'smudge sticks' made from bundles of sage to cleanse and clear negative energy. Physically, it has a calming effect on the nervous system, can clear headaches, aid respiratory problems, and relieve other stress-related conditions.

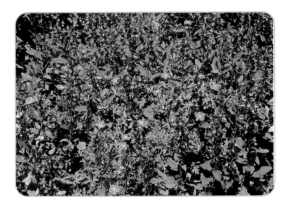

Sage (*Salvia officinalis*)

St John's wort

Found throughout the British Isles, St John's wort or *Hypericum perforatum* has small yellow flowers and black spotted leaves. Its flowers are harvested and dried for their natural ingredient, hypericum. The name 'hypericum' is derived from the Greek words *hyper* (above) and *eikon* (picture) in reference to its traditional use of warding off evil, by hanging the plant over a picture in the house on St John's Day, 24 June. The species name *perforatum* derives from the small holes in the leaves, which can be seen when they are held against the light.

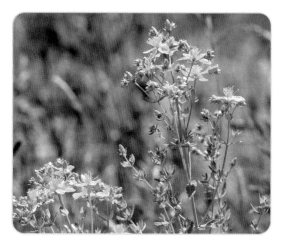

St John's wort (*Hypericum perforatum*)

A study quoted in the *Evening Standard's* Metro Magazine (11 February 2005), comparing the effectiveness of St John's wort with the anti-depressant drug paroxetine (also known as Serotax), reported that 'It is as effective an anti-depressant as prescription drugs . . . half the patients treated with St John's wort felt less depressed after six weeks but only a third of sufferers on paroxetine improved over the same period . . . the study of 224 people with moderate to severe depression also suggested St John's wort was less likely to cause side effects such as stomach aches.' St John's wort raises serotonin and dopamine levels – the 'feel good hormones' – and it is widely used today as a natural anti-depressant. It promotes healing and has a restorative effect on the nervous system; it is also used to treat stress, anxiety, sleep disorders and tension headaches.

When taken in oral form, St John's wort is known to cause certain medications to metabolise through the body too quickly, thereby decreasing their effectiveness. These include other antidepressants, the oral contraceptive pill, blood-thinning and cholesterol-lowering medications. Its oral form is also contraindicated during pregnancy. Clients on any medications (including over-the-counter) are advised to consult their pharmacist or doctor prior to taking any product containing St John's wort. However, as it is not taken in oral form, the manufacturers do not list the tiny amount used in ear candles as a contraindication, but if you have any doubts you should seek professional advice or choose ear candles without this ingredient.

Essential oils

Some ear candles combine traditional
constituents with essential oils, which are
concentrated organic substance, obtained
from plant life. Essential oils are present in
tiny amounts in a large number of plants,
and they are often referred to as the 'life
force' or 'hormone' of the plant. They are
'essential' to plant life and play an important
role in a plant's metabolism; eg they protect
against disease, have anti-bacterial qualities
and their aroma attracts or repels certain
animals/insects. The scent of a flower, herb
or spice is due to its essential oil content.

Essential oils are quite different from fatty
oils, and have a consistency more like water
than oil. Their chemistry is complex and they
are highly volatile. They all have a unique
smell and unique therapeutic qualities.

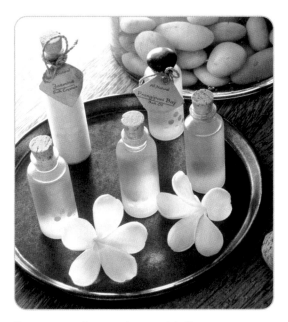

Some ear candles contain essential oils

Types of ear candles

There are several types of ear candles
available on the market. One of the market
leaders is a German company called Biosun,
which was founded in 1984. In 1985 they
made contact with the traditional Hopi
Indians, and through meetings with
traditional Hopi elders they developed ear
candles based on the traditional herbal
formula, but using cotton rather than leaves
as was the Hopi practice. There are also
several types of 'basic' candles, as well as ear
cones marketed under various trade names.

Factors affecting choice of candles

- size and shape
- constituents
- safety features
- comfort.

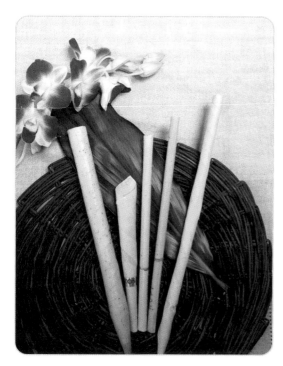

A variety of ear candles

Size and shape

Candles can be cylindrical or cone-shaped and vary in diameter and length. The end of the candle to be inserted into the ear can be tapered or flat-ended. The candle seam can either be spiral or straight. The size and shape of a candle will largely determine the comfort for the user and how long it takes to burn.

Constituents

Some candles are simply made from cotton, cotton-flax or hemp and sprayed with beeswax. Others have the added benefit of being infused with ingredients such honey and herbs. The herbs traditionally used were chosen for their benefit to the ear, nose and throat area and their ability to stimulate the immune system. Candle colour varies according to the quality of the beeswax and the constituents used.

Safety features

Products displaying a 'CE' mark are certified medical products according to medical device directive 93/42/EEC, and have undergone rigorous testing in regard to quality and safety. Some form of filter should be incorporated into the candle design to prevent hot wax or other ingredients falling into the client's ear during the treatment.

A safety marker line on the lower end of the candle indicates when the candle should be extinguished. Candles should be supplied in a sealed bag or container with information about the ingredients and clear instructions on their use. Candles should be stored away from heat and out of direct sunlight to enable them to keep their shape. However if they do become a bit squashed, they can easily be reshaped.

Comfort

It is important that the client is comfortable during the treatment so that they can relax and enjoy the experience. The actual 'candles' used in modern therapeutic treatments (such as those manufactured by Biosun) are cylindrical, ensuring that no sharp points can be inserted into clients' ears. For children or adult clients with a very small entrance to the ear canal, Otosan ear cones may be more comfortable. The safety features such as 'maximum burn' line also ensure that the radiating heat from the candle does not cause any discomfort to the client.

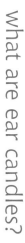

Hopi ear candles

The most popular are Biosun's cylindrical candles, which have been on the market for over twenty years. They are around 22cm long with a diameter of 8mm and a burning time of 10–12 minutes. Constituents are cotton, pure beeswax, honey extract and traditional herbs such as sage, St John's wort, and chamomile. A range of candles with pure essential oils is also available.

Safety features include the red or green line (maximum burn line) around the candle and a specially developed safety filter to ensure simple and safe application. They are flat-ended rather than pointed so that the candle cannot be pushed too far into the ear (the curved shape of the ear canal also prevents this). They have a straight seam to enable the user to influence where ash may fall (ie away from the face), as when the candle burns, the ash falls back from the seam. Biosun ear candles are regularly tested by independent institutes and are registered as medical products class IIa according to Medical Device Directive 93/42/EEC.

Ear cones

There are several varieties of cone-shaped ear candles on the market. The market leader in ear cones is an Italian company called Otosan whose ear cones are compliant with EU regulation 93/42/EEC regarding safety and quality. They are wider at the top and shorter than traditional Hopi ear candles. Safety features of Otosan ear cones include a protective disc to protect the ear and head area from heat and any possibility of burning fragments, as well as a flame-breaking ring that automatically extinguishes the flame at the end of the treatment. They also feature a valve rather than a filter, which ensures that the upward movement of air is not impeded, as well as preventing any candle material from

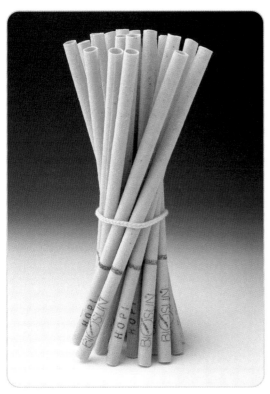

Biosun ear candles

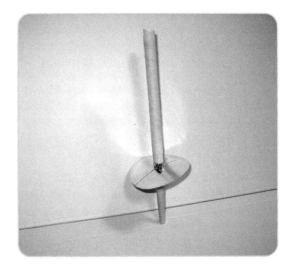

An Otosan ear cone

dripping into the ear. This makes them easy, safe and practical to use, and with a shorter burning time of five to seven minutes, they are suitable for the treatment of children or clients who may not have time for a longer session.

Constituents are cotton, beeswax, paraffin wax and propolis. Otosan also produce oil-based ear drops enriched with propolis and herbs, which are excellent for soothing irritation in the ear canal or around the ear area.

Basic candles

These are usually marketed as 'natural ear candles' and are purely candles (cotton flax or hemp with beeswax) with no other ingredients added, although some manufacturers add essential oils and herbs, which will be listed. The majority are made in the USA or Canada. The cotton or hemp is generally organically grown and unbleached, and the beeswax locally sourced.

There is a large variety available on the market. Their size and shape vary, and their burning time will depend on this. They generally have no specialised safety features, so the manufacturer's instructions need to be carefully followed. They do provide a cheaper alternative to the market leaders. Many of these candles are very large and some manufacturers advise the use of one candle to treat both ears. In such cases it is necessary to burn the candle down to a marker, carefully extinguish it, and then cut the end before relighting it and inserting it into the other ear.

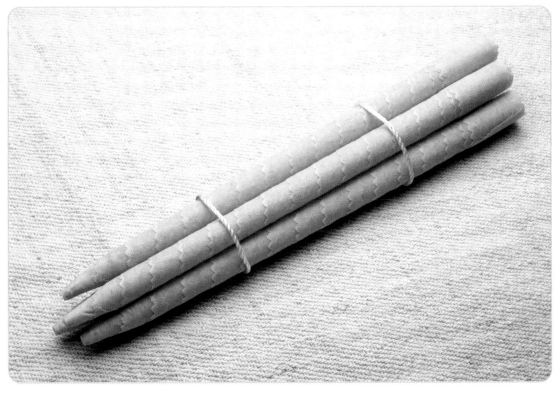

Some basic 'natural' ear candles

FAQs

Is it safe to use ear candles that contain paraffin wax or soybean wax?

Paraffin is a byproduct in the petroleum refining chain and emits high levels of toxic chemicals that include lead benzene (the same as from your car exhaust pipe) and acetone, both known to be carcinogenic. When burned, paraffin wax creates a lot of soot, which pollutes indoor air and lungs; in our opinion, inhaling toxic waste cannot be therapeutic. Some candles are made using purified paraffin wax or man-made food grade paraffin, the same kind used in coating cheese and chocolate to make it look shiny. They burn quite cleanly but do not have the therapeutic value of beeswax.

Soy ear candles come from a vegetable (soy bean), are non-toxic, do not produce soot, are 100 per cent biodegradable, burn 50 per cent longer and at a lower temperature than paraffin. However, a large proportion of the soy bean harvest today is either genetically modified (GMO) or non-GMO mixed in with GMO soy beans.

Can I use ear candles containing pre-blended essential oils if I am not an aromatherapist?

Since you are not blending the oils yourself and the manufacturers will have ensured that the essential oils are present at a safe limit, you can use candles containing pre-blended essential oils. There are con-traindications to certain essential oils used in aromatherapy treatments. However, as the oils are present in tiny amounts in the candles, the manufacturers do not currently advise contraindications with regard to the essential oil content. Any doubts should be checked with the manufacturers.

Is it safe to use ear candles that do not have a filter?

The purpose of the filter is to prevent residue from the ear candle falling into the ear. When you open up a Biosun ear candle, you can see that this residue remains above the filter, and if the filter were not present this could end up in the ear canal. Some insurers will not cover you to use basic ear candles that do not conform to EU safety regulations.

For candles that do not have a filter, some manufacturers recommend cutting a small piece of medical gauze and pushing it to about a quarter of the way up the candle from the base (below the maximum burn line). However, this may disrupt the air flow a little, but will be safer than using a candle with no filter.

What are Canadian ear candles?

These are a variety of natural ear candles imported from Canada. They are made with pure cotton and beeswax produced locally to the manufacturer and usually contain no other additives, although some do contain herbs which should be listed. The ends are tapered and slightly rounded to ensure they sit comfortably in the ear. They are generally about 10 inches (25.5 cm) long and 1/2 inches (1.27 cm) wide. As with all ear candles the treatment should ideally be carried out by someone who has been instructed in their use.

how ear candles work

Ear candling has a consistent record of success in promoting positive health, and there is much speculation on the question, 'how does it work?' Some people even find it amusing that a 'candle' to promote health is placed in a person's ear. How can a simple ear candle achieve so much?

The fact that ear candling has a rich and ancient history in many cultures indicates that it is a powerful healing tool, as useful today as it was in former times. Modern research has proven what the ancients instinctively knew – that it works on a physical, emotional and subtle energy level, and we will look at these aspects.

Physical

Gentle massaging and suction effects

Being a hollow tube or cone, the centre of an ear candle is simply a column of air rather than a solid mass. When lit at the top, the rising air column inside the candle begins to heat up. As the candle burns down, it continues to heat up the top of the rising air column in the centre of the candle. The rising air column creates a very mild suction action at the base, which helps to loosen compacted earwax.

At the same time, the beeswax and other ingredients (which are infused in the fabric of the tube or cone) are vapourised. These ingredients, some of which are slightly oily, make some of the air inside the candle heavier and it spirals downwards into the ear canal, setting up pressure waves and gentle sound waves from the sizzling ingredients, which massage the eardrum. Since even the slightest movement of the eardrum is carried onwards to the middle and inner ear, all of the structures of the ear receive a gentle massage. As the ear, nose, sinuses and throat are all interconnected, this has the effect of regulating and balancing pressure in the ears as well as the whole of the upper respiratory

19

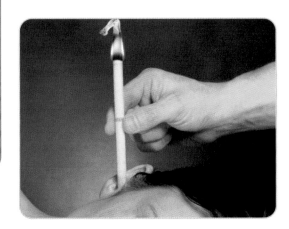

A Biosun ear candle alight

The intact eardrum prevents the vapours from travelling any further than the outer ear; however, it is speculated that some molecules may diffuse across the membrane. No vacuum is created, otherwise the receiver would be unable to hear the sizzling sound of the ingredients burning down. In any event, a vacuum could be potentially damaging to the eardrum.

Contrary to what some people say, no earwax or anything else is 'sucked up' out of the ear canal, as the suction effect is very slight. Laboratory analysis of the post-treatment residue showed that 'no ear wax, skin cells or hairs were detected' (Sceats, 2004). In opening up an ear candle after treatment, it is clear to see that any residue found in the ear candle is always above and never below the filter, so it would be impossible for this to be anything other than beeswax and powder from the ear candle itself. This same residue can be found

tract. Users often describe a soothing, light sensation in the ear and head area as the sinuses are drained and cleared. Clearer nasal breathing and an improved sense of smell (even when the nose was blocked before treatment) are often experienced, as well as a wonderful feeling of relaxation.

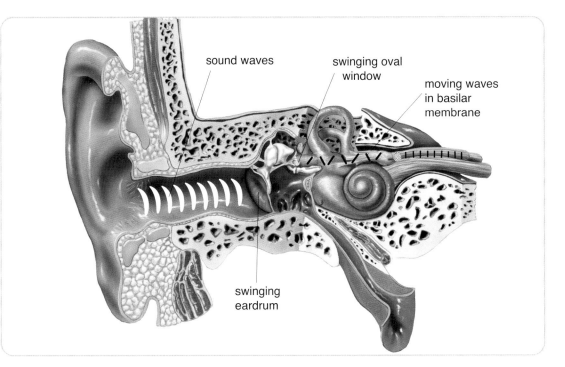

sound waves

swinging oval window

moving waves in basilar membrane

swinging eardrum

Sound and pressure waves massage the eardrum

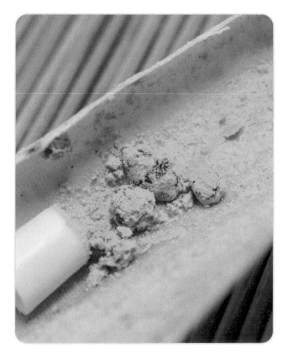

Ear candle residue remains above the filter

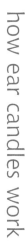

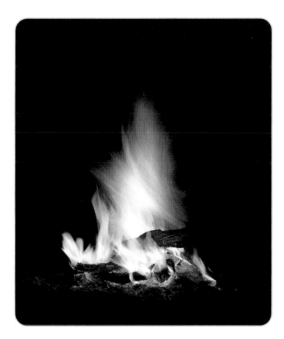

reduction of endogenic stress factors' found that 'the physical variations in air pressure within the tube caused by the combustion process have a pressure compensatory effect on the eardrum and promote secretion in the frontal and paranasal sinuses. At the same time important energy points and reflex zones are stimulated.' Several of the major energy meridians (see page 27) have points close to the ear and the ear itself is rich in reflex points. A diagrams of these 'acupoints' is shown on page 77.

Heat

Just as you do not need to sit right on top of an open fire to feel the heat, so the heat from the flame of the candle radiates outwards in all directions, warming up the surrounding air. As it burns downwards and the flame becomes closer to the ear, this radiating heat becomes stronger. The location of the safety

by simply burning an ear candle down without inserting it into an ear, allowing it to cool and opening it. In our experience (but not clinically proven) the varying amounts of residue found above the filter may reflect the condition of the ears and associated structures, with more residues normally remaining when problems are more severe. Problems such as compacted earwax may decrease the space for the vapours to circulate, and problems with other parts of the ears and related structures may sap the heat energy from the candle rather than allowing it to be used in burning off the ingredients. In most cases we have found that severe conditions result in more residue remaining after treatment.

A report published by Biosun Scientific Advisory Council on the use of ear candles by medical doctors in the treatment of 'diseases in the region of the ear and head, as well as the

The radiant heat of an open fire

marker line on Biosun ear candles indicates the point at which you should remove the candle from the ear so that the heat does not become uncomfortable. The location of this line was arrived at after rigorous testing to ensure the comfort and safety of the receiver. Otosan ear cones incorporate a 'flame-breaking' safety ring, indicating this point.

Although the vapours inside the hollow tube are slightly warm, at no time does the base of the ear candle (which rests at the entrance to the ear canal) become hot, because the temperature of the vapour-filled air inside the candle drops as it moves away from the flame.

Another element which generates heat is the presence of the therapist's hand as it supports the candle in the ear, close to the face of the receiver. German naturopathic doctors who regularly use Biosun ear candles in the treatment of tinnitus have stated that 'the locally applied warmth stimulates vascularisation, invigorates the immune system and reinforces the flow of lymph.' (1998) The heat, along with the hydrating effects of the vapours, helps to soften and loosen compacted earwax, which can be expelled up to 48 hours after a treatment. It is usually expelled naturally in the shower or on the pillow in the morning.

Vapours

Many of the constituents of the candles have properties that calm and soothe the nervous system, and also have the effect of lifting depression and promoting a 'feel-good factor'. While the ear candles are burning, the

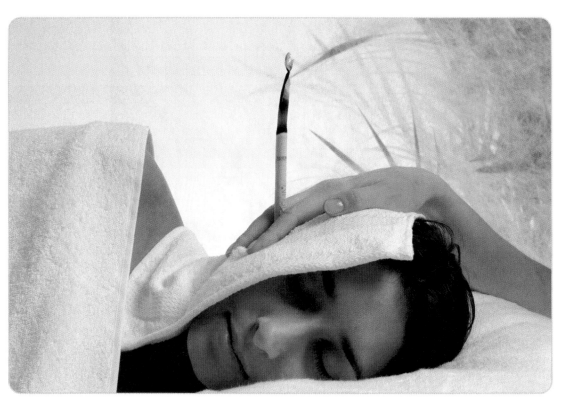

The warmth of the therapist's hand soothes the ear area

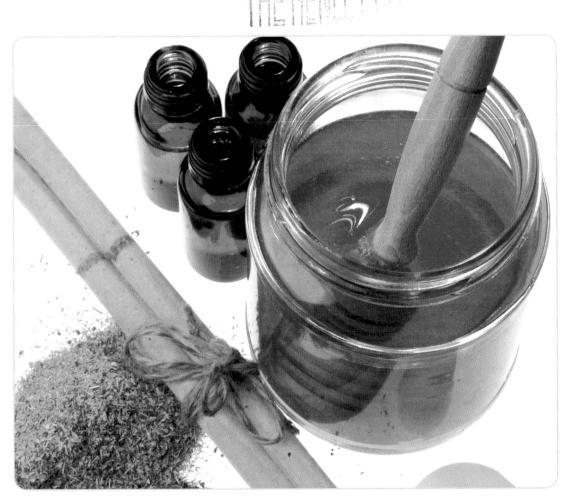

The vapourised ingredients calm and soothe the nervous system

ingredients are vapourised and some of the molecules trigger the olfactory nerve, which sends signals to the brain. On the roof of each nasal cavity there are roughly ten million olfactory receptor cells with six to eight tiny sensory hairs (cilia) projecting from each cell. These cells are unique in that they are replaced every 30 days, unlike other nerve cells in the body which are not replaced when damaged. Odour molecules from the ear candles float back into the nasal cavity where they are absorbed by the receptor cells, which fire impulses to the smell centre in the brain, only an inch away. This ancient, mysterious

part of the brain, known as the limbic system, is associated with memories and emotions. Some odour molecules are inhaled into the lungs where they are absorbed into the bloodstream and carried all around the body.

Touch

Touch is essential for healthy physical and emotional development, and many studies exist which demonstrate its power and importance. A famous experiment carried out by psychologist Harry Harlow on rhesus macaque monkeys (which share roughly 94 per cent of their genetic heritage with humans) in the late 1950s demonstrated that touch is even more important than food. A group of baby monkeys was taken from their real mother and put in a cage with a fake nursing 'mother' made from wire mesh with milk bottles instead of breasts. The babies were fed but not touched or held, and they soon began to show signs of trauma and depression. Another soft cloth mother with an empty breast and a sweet smile was introduced and within days, all signs of trauma disappeared as the baby monkeys snuggled up to the to the cloth surrogate, only darting quickly to and from the wire mesh mother when they were hungry.

At the Touch Research Institute (TRI) in Miami, Florida, founded by Tiffany Field, researchers examining the effects of touch have demonstrated that it has anxiety-reducing, calming and relaxing effects on children and adults. TRI has conducted more than 90 studies on the positive effects of touch therapy on many medical conditions. Among the significant findings are enhanced growth (premature babies), diminished pain (fibro-myalgia), decreased autoimmune problems, enhanced immune function (increased natural killer cells in HIV and cancer), and enhanced alertness and performance.

The major cause for improvement in these conditions is decreased levels of stress hormones. A hormone called oxytocin, released through touch, lowers levels of stress hormones. In 1906, an English researcher Sir Henry Dale discovered a substance in the pituitary gland that could speed up the birthing process. Later, he found that it also promotes the expression of breast milk. He named it oxytocin, from the Greek words for 'quick childbirth labour.' Oxytocin was later shown to play a physiological role, particularly in calming patients, and is able to influence many vital functions in the body. In

hospital settings, older patients who receive massage sleep better, experience less pain, need less medication and sometimes become less confused and more sociable, probably due to increased oxytocin and endorphin levels. Although we normally associate this hormone with childbirth because it is produced in vast amounts in response to uterine contractions, both females and males have the same distribution of oxytocin-producing cells. It is possible to elevate levels of oxytocin in both men and women with a combination of stimuli, such as warmth, touch and massage.

The good news is that it is not only the person on the receiving end of 'touch therapy' that benefits from oxytocin release. Studies show that the person administering 'touch' also experiences heightened levels of oxytocin. According to Kerstin Uvnas Moberg, author of *The Oxytocin Factor* (2003), many massage therapists exhibit the effects of high levels of oxytocin, such as lower levels of stress hormones and lowered blood pressure.

It has been scientifically proven that touch releases endorphins in the body. Endorphins literally means 'endogenous morphine' or morphine produced within the body. Morphine is a drug which produces euphoric effects and kills pain. In her book *Molecules of Emotion* (1997), neuroscientist Candace Pert details her research on how the chemicals in the human body form a dynamic information network, linking mind and body. She states: 'from my research with endorphins, I know the power of touch to stimulate and regulate our natural chemicals, the ones that are tailored to act at precisely the right times in exactly the appropriate doses to maximise our feelings of health and wellbeing.' This is one of the reasons why clients often experience pain relief after any form of touch therapy.

Ear candling is a gentle but powerful touch therapy, and the effects of the treatment can be further enhanced by a specialised massage of the face, neck, ears and scalp. The treatment can have a significant effect on balancing mind and body and giving a feeling of wellbeing.

casestudy

The following anecdotes sent to us by practitioners Penny and Linda clearly demonstrate the endorphin effects of the treatment.

Penny writes: 'My son Stephen, aged 22, had an accident at work resulting in several severely broken bones including his right femur. He is a very active person and was finding it extremely difficult to relax, so I decided to try Hopi ear candling as he has always enjoyed this treatment. As the candles were burning down, I noticed that the flame on the right side burnt very brightly, and on the left side it burnt as normal. Both candles took 12 minutes to burn down. When I opened the candle that was used on the right ear, I found the wax residue, extending to almost two inches, looked exactly like a skeletal leg including a thickening where the femur was damaged! Stephen said the pains in his leg had improved. He had several subsequent ear candling treatments and some reiki, and the hospital doctors were amazed by his speedy recovery.'

Linda writes of her own experience: 'A 51-year-old woman went on an ear candling course on a Friday, suffering at the time with a lot of indeterminate knee pain which had been going on for several months. Over the following weekend she noticed that the pain had virtually gone, and now only comes back for short periods intermittently. Strange, but true!'

Subtle energy

Auras and chakras

Man has a subtle energy field that coexists with the physical body, often referred to as the aura, which permeates the physical body and extends outwards, surrounding the body. Energy within the aura is given different names in different cultures, eg *chi* in China, *ki* in Japan and *prana* in India. In the West it is known as the 'life-force', for it is said to be the universal energy that sustains all living things. Western Christianity shows this energy as a halo surrounding the crown of the head, usually depicted on saints and angels. Just as the physical body has an anatomical structure, so does the aura. The size of the aura depends on the level of development of the individual; a large aura indicates a higher level of development.

Within the aura are seven major energy centres called chakras. Chakra is a Sanskrit word meaning 'wheel of light'. Chakras are traditionally thought of as spinning vortices of energy that are located at different levels from the base of the spine to the crown of the head, permeating the physical body and

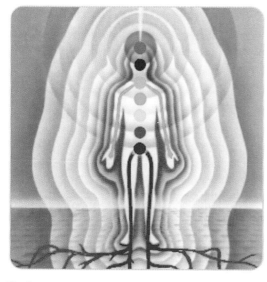

The human aura

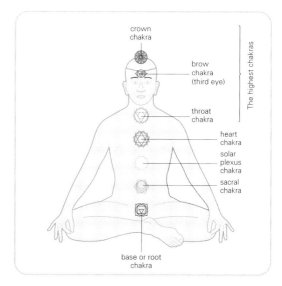

The seven major chakras

extending into the aura. Each chakra forms a specific layer of the aura. Secondary chakras are located in the palms of the hands and the soles of the feet. Chakras are gateways for the flow of energy and life into the physical body, and the means through which the physical body communicates with the aura. To the ancients, chakra knowledge was an important part of life, and this knowledge has survived through ancient texts.

The chakras vibrate at a different frequency, from the lower slower frequency in the base chakra, increasing through the chakras to the higher faster frequency in the crown chakra. Each chakra relates to an organ and gland of the body, and to a unique area of human experience. Traditionally, each chakra has an element and colour associated with it (the colours form those of a rainbow):

	Chakra	Element	Colour	Physical body	Human experience
1	Base	Earth	Red	Spine, kidneys, adrenals	Survival, security, confidence, strength
2	Sacral	Water	Orange	Reproductive, spleen, bladder	Sexual energy, emotions
3	Solar plexus	Fire	Yellow	Liver, stomach, pancreas	Power and wisdom
4	Heart	Air	Green	Heart, thymus	Love, compassion
5	Throat	Ether	Blue	Lungs, throat, thyroid and parathyroid	Communication, creativity, self-expression
6	Third eye	Mind	Indigo	Brain, pineal	Intuition, knowledge
7	Crown	Spirit	Violet	Brain, pituitary	Spiritual aspiration

The lower three chakras – base, sacral and solar plexus – relate to the physical plane, whereas the higher three chakras – throat, third eye and crown – relate to communication, knowledge and the spiritual realm. The fourth chakra – the heart – is a bridge between the lower and higher charkas, and relates to love and compassion.

Everyday activities affect chakra energy, as this subtle energy is dynamic and constantly changing. It changes in response to diet, emotions, exercise, stress, injuries and healing work. Simply having negative thoughts depletes chakra energy, whereas positive thoughts help to heal and energise. Suppressed emotions such as fear, hurt, grief and anger are held within the aura and cause stagnant energy in the chakras. On a physical level, this can lead to tiredness, a lowered immune system and eventually illness; on an emotional level this can lead to feelings of disharmony, isolation and the inability to give or receive love. Each chakra is connected, and an imbalance in one will affect the others.

The meridians

Energy travels through the physical body, flowing in lines called meridians which act as pathways for energy between the chakras and the organs they relate to. In Chinese medicine, the key to health is a balanced meridian flow that carries chi throughout the body. An acupuncturist stimulates certain points on the meridians to promote the flow of energy along the meridians, bringing harmony to the subtle energy that in turn promotes healing to the physical body and the emotional state. Knowledge of chakras and

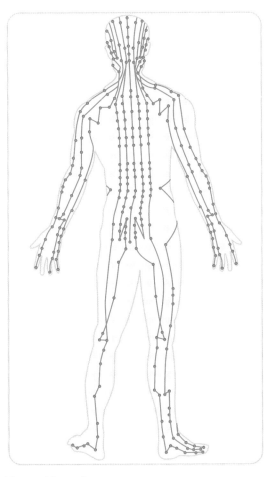

The meridians of acupuncture

meridians helps experts in different disciplines to obtain a more holistic view of the human body. The ear is mapped with acupuncture points (acupoints) of the entire body, in the shape of an upside-down foetus, and is a gateway to the whole of the meridian system. The acupoints of the ears can be stimulated by massage of the ears. See Chapter 7 for further information and a diagram of the acupoints of the ear on page 77.

27

How ear candling works on the subtle energy

Many healing modalities and exercise regimes strive to achieve healing and harmony to man's subtle energy, eg homeopathy, reiki, tai chi, and yoga. The simple ear candle also has an effect on subtle energy. For our research on this book, we used Kirlian photography to check the electro-magnetic energy field of clients before and after treatments, and we observed changes in the before and after photographs. We have included an example here. We also used clairvoyant observation of the aura during ear candling treatments. This research confirmed that ear candling works on a very deep level.

Kirlian photography

The study of energy and healing is of significant importance, and the use of Kirlian photography has the ability to show the vibrations of the electromagnetic field, which surrounds all living things. The way in which this energy field vibrates indicates a person's health at every level. The process of Kirlian photography is named after Seymon Kirlian, a Russian inventor who pioneered the first efforts on the process in the 1930s as a means of visualising the electro-magnetic fields around living things. Each time we move, think or respond emotionally to something, we produce tiny pulses of electrical energy. The Kirlian camera uses electron cascades to make this subtle energy visible, in a similar way that iron filings can make magnetic fields around magnets visible. Any part of the energy field monitored can give a meaningful picture of the whole. Kirlian photography uses the hands as the electromagnetic energy field is particularly strong around the hands – they are the sites of secondary chakras, and there is an abundance

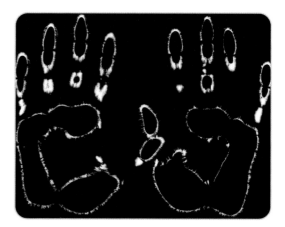

Kirlian photograph 1: taken before an ear candling treatment

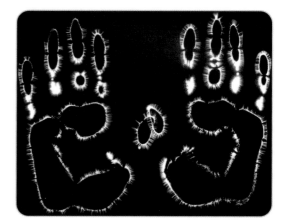

Kirlian photograph 2: taken after an ear candling treatment

of nerve endings in the fingers. In Kirlian photography the vibration of the energy field is shown as an image of each hand; size, shape and density indicate its vibration.

Photograph 1 above displays the patterns created by the electromagnetic field before an ear candling treatment. The individual presented with a stress-related headache. Gaps in the image indicate energy blocks in the electromagnetic field, such as on the right hand below the tip of the ring finger. In this case, the gap relates to creative action being blocked by lack of confidence and self-doubt. Photograph 2 was taken after an ear candling treatment. This image is denser and has more vibrancy; there is now no gap below the tip of the right finger, indicating an increased energy level and a rising of creative power. After the treatment, the individual reported that her headache had subsided and she felt a relaxed state of mind and increased energy levels.

Clairvoyance

In looking at a human being, most of us just see the physical body, but a sensitised eye – a clairvoyant – can see the aura, composed of various layers of energy and colours that surround the physical body. The condition of the aura is perceived in terms of size, colour, vibrancy and density. It is often said that ear candling can have an effect on the aura, so we were interested to investigate this further. We sought the services of a respected clairvoyant who made observations during ear candling treatments, and below is an extract from her observations.

Our research gives credence to the ancient use of ear candling and scented herbs to cleanse and clear negative energy, and to the shamanic belief that 'fire releases that part of yourself which no longer serves you' – see Chapter 1.

casestudy

'In each case, the effects on the aura were immediate, and each client's aura responded in a unique way, depending on where the weaknesses were. The energy of the base chakra responded to ear candling by sending energy upward through the chakra system to the crown, enhancing the flow of energy along the meridian lines. This movement of energy resulted in the chakras being calmed and revitalised. There was a release and purification of stagnant energy associated with negative emotions such as anger, hurt and resentment, the ear canal serving as a point of release of stagnant energy. This energy change was seen to have a specific action on parts of the body such as the liver, kidneys, heart, spleen, gall bladder, and throat as well as on glands such as the pituitary, pineal, hypothalamus and thymus.

'At the last stages of the treatment, the third eye and crown chakras on all clients observed assumed a much quieter vibration – they were stiller and at peace and working together in harmony, promoting clarity and an increased mental faculty. This clearing and strengthening of chakra energy promotes a raised immune system and positive health on all levels.

'For one male client, the solar plexus chakra was spinning in the wrong direction before treatment, and in the first few minutes of the treatment I observed it change to spin in the correct direction (which is anticlockwise) and a normal energy pattern connected. This calmed and connected the centre of the auric field, harmonised the client and "quietened" his stress. As a healer myself, I was surprised at how effective the ear candling treatment is. I feel that deep energy blocks may require a course of treatments to facilitate significant improvement.'

FAQs

Does the effect of ear candling vary depending on the type of candle used?
The basic principles of how ear candles work are the same for all types of candles. The effects vary, depending on the constituents of the candles.

Does ear candling affect the therapist's aura, as well as the client's?
During our research it was observed that the therapist's energy field reacted positively during treatments. This is due to the therapist's proximity to the flame of the candle, the inhalation of the scented herbs and the positive response of the body to touch.

Can I do ear candling on myself?
We do not recommend doing the treatment on yourself, as it is very relaxing and you may fall asleep and burn yourself. You will obtain much more benefit by allowing yourself to completely relax and enjoy the treatment administered by someone else.

the benefits of ear candling

As a complementary therapy, ear candling does not claim to cure any disorders. However, therapists who carry out this treatment all agree that one of its most marked effects on their clients is a feeling of total relaxation. When the body reaches this state, many positive health benefits result. The parasympathetic nervous system is stimulated, leading to lowered heart and respiratory rates and increased peristalsis in the digestive system. This state of relaxation produces positive healing chemicals in the body and is an antidote to the harmful chemicals produced when the body is under constant stress. There is much anecdotal evidence showing the positive effects of ear candling, and hopefully more empirical evidence will become available as complementary therapists are encouraged to carry out research in the course of their work.

Biosun who manufacture the traditional Hopi ear candles have pioneered some clinical studies, one of which was carried out by medical professionals between February

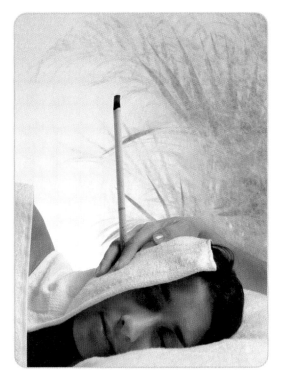

A client receiving an ear candling treatment

31

and June 2000. In 11 test centres, 78 patients (30 males and 48 females) suffering from colds, tinnitus, headaches, secondary effects of colds, headaches and stress symptoms such as insomnia and anxiety, were hospitalised to observe the effects of Biosun ear candles in treating their conditions. Some symptoms were acute and some chronic, while some patients had multiple symptoms. The age range was from 3 to 91 years, with an average age of 43 years. The length of treatment ranged from one to 75 days, with an average of 23 days. The average application was nine treatments per patient, with one patient receiving 15 treatments and one patient receiving a single treatment.

With all the patients, there was a decrease in the symptoms during the course of the treatments, with acute conditions becoming less severe to the point of no complaints, and chronic conditions becoming milder. In the overall efficacy assessment, 93.3 per cent of investigators and 89.7 per cent of patients gave a verdict of 'very good' or 'good'. Full details of this study are available from Biosun (see Useful Addresses on p 101).

In 1992, a magazine published by the Centre of Natural Medicine in Milan reported the results of a number of tests carried out by a group of doctors on the use of the Otosan ear cone. They found that the cones worked effectively with no contraindications or side effects, and were a good natural alternative to local analgesics. 'In the first case 15 adults were tested. They presented with an abundance of earwax, or the actual formation of a plug, and complained of itchiness, difficulty in perceiving sounds, buzzing and hissing sounds. After the cone had been applied, all patients reported an immediate improvement of their symptoms, and when examined using an otoscope a decrease in wax could be observed.

'In the second case, 15 schoolchildren suffering from otalgia (earache) who had not taken pain-killers for at least six hours were considered. Most of the children reported a remarkable reduction in pain after only five minutes from the end of the treatment with the cone. At a test carried out two hours later, the pain had not returned. As a result of these tests, doctors have formed a positive judgement on the use of the Otosan cone.'

In Germany in 1995, a television programme entitled 'An hour in the doctor's surgery' was broadcast containing some interviews on the use of ear cones. Among the interviewees, Mrs Ulrike Lorbiezki said: 'I use ear cones on my children as a supplementary remedy against heavy colds and flu. Especially Tassilo who is five and has a particular tendency for colds followed by inflammation of the lateral cavities and of the ears. I always use the cones on both ears when the cold persists and begins to settle into the nose. I carry out the treatment before putting them to bed, because I have noticed that the children sleep more peacefully during the night. In this way I cure the cold using fewer drugs.' In the course of the same programme, Klaus Krieg, a homeopath, stated that he applies the cones also to patients suffering from headaches, migraine, sinusitis, neuralgia and pains resulting from stress. Mr Jungfer, one of Krieg's patients, said: 'About three years ago I used to hear buzzing in my ears. I always had a strange sensation and woke up during the night. I went to the doctor, had x-rays done, but I wasn't satisfied with the results because symptoms persisted. Ever since Dr Krieg treated me with ear cones problems have disappeared. The therapy is effective and today I still undergo treatment every four weeks.' Further details of the benefits of ear cones are available from Otosan (see Where to go from here chapter, p 102).

Ear candling is carried out with the client fully clothed, and so appeals to those who may feel embarrassed about undressing.

The treatment generally includes a massage of the face, neck, scalp and ears. This adds to the beneficial effects of the treatment as it stimulates the circulation of blood carrying oxygen and nutrients to the tissues and encourages the elimination of waste through the blood and lymphatic system. The treatment has proven to be effective for various ailments.

Bell's palsy

Bell's palsy occurs because of injury and inflammation of the facial nerve (seventh cranial nerve) which produces paralysis of the facial muscles. The injury may be caused by pressure on the nerve due to a tumour, inner ear infection, meningitis, high blood pressure, or dental surgery. It is also associated with the cold sore virus (herpes simplex virus). There is a drooping of the mouth on the affected side, with the eyes remaining open even during sleep and a loss of taste sensations. Corticosteroids are usually prescribed to

reduce the inflammation. Colds and chills can trigger Bell's palsy, and the gentle heat generated by the candle combined with the anti-inflammatory effects of some of the ingredients can aid in the healing process. When the inflammation has died down, the face massage can° help increase muscle tone on the affected side and stimulate the paralysed muscles. Facial exercises and gentle face massage at home can continue the healing process. Most cases of Bell's palsy make a complete recovery.

Candidiasis or candida

This is a yeast overgrowth that is normally associated with the vaginal or oral area (commonly called thrush), but it can invade and affect the whole body. Triggers include antibiotics, long-term stress and diets high in sugar. There are many symptoms including itching which can affect the ear canal, a dark, damp place where fungal infections can

thrive. Avoidance of sugary and yeast-containing foods and drinks is recommended. The vapourised ingredients in the ear candles can help to soothe the ear canal and alleviate the itching associated with this condition, but treatment should not be carried out if any inflammation or infection is present.

33

Colds

Colds can occur at any time of year, although they are more frequent in the colder months. About 50 per cent of the British population develop at least one cold per year. Symptoms include frequent sneezing, runny nose, sore throat, cough and sometimes bacterial ear infections, which travel up through the Eustachian tube from the throat. Ear candling will not cure a cold but can help clear congestion and ease discomfort. The candles can be used every second or third day during the first week of a cold, and then every three days in the second week if symptoms persist. Therapists should not treat while the client is actively coughing and sneezing.

Earaches

Earaches can have many causes, including outer ear infections (otitis externa), middle ear infections (otitis media) or inner ear infections (otitis interna). The cause should be investigated and diagnosed by a doctor. Just as aches and pains can often be eased by placing a hot water bottle on the area, the gentle heat radiating from the candle, the warm vapours and the heat from the therapist's hand close to the ear can help to alleviate some earaches. In cases of otitis externa, an inflammation of the ear canal (usually caused by infection or allergy), treatment is not recommended as it would be too uncomfortable for the client. In this case, treatment with ear drops may be effective.

Excessive ear wax

Ear wax can sometimes build up in the outer ear canal and impact on the eardrum, leading to temporary hearing loss and a general feeling of discomfort. Ear candling can be used as a natural alternative to orthodox treatments such as cotton swabs, metal scrapers and syringing with water, which are all quite invasive and can damage the eardrum. As the candle burns, the spiralling smoke travels into the outer ear canal, gently warming the ear, while massage improves the efficiency of the temporomandibular joint which helps to move wax away from the eardrum. When the wax is softened, it loosens and expands; this can result in an increase in hearing loss before the wax is gradually expelled, usually within 48 hours of treatment. Several treatments may be necessary before an improvement is seen. Regular treatments every six to eight weeks may help to prevent excessive wax build-up.

casestudy

Practitioner Gurjit treated Mandip, aged 25, for ear problems:

'Mandip is 25 and has had ear problems from birth; her tonsils were removed at the age of 9, and she had grommets inserted while at school. She has constant problems with her ears, and syringing does not work for her, even though the doctor has said that her ears are full of hard wax. She is hard of hearing in her left ear as a result, and attributes frequent headaches and poor sleep patterns to the build-up of wax. She has made suggested changes to her diet such as giving up dairy products, but this made no difference. I treated her once a week for three weeks initially, and now give her a treatment at her request once a fortnight. Each time the results are the same: wax residue is plentiful and quite hard. She finds that a few days after each treatment, when she cleans her ears, the wax is looser.

Mandip is quite a nervous person regarding treatments, and it is impossible to give her an Indian head massage treatment as she fidgets and does not relax, however hard I try. But despite being nervous at her first ear candling treatment, she now drifts off to sleep very quickly and loves the face massage. She dislikes having her ears syringed, and feels that ear candling loosens the earwax and is much less invasive and uncomfortable. Some of my other clients find this a relaxing treatment and have reported sleeping better and experiencing the natural removal of earwax after a treatment.'

Glue ear

Glue ear (secretory otitis media) is an increasingly common childhood disorder in which a viscous fluid accumulates in the middle ear. The sticky glue-like fluid prevents the ossicles from vibrating, leading to deafness. It is caused by a malfunction of the Eustachian tube, which does not open as it should in response to swallowing and yawning. This causes a vacuum in the middle ear, leading to inflammation and the production of fluid, which gradually thickens. It can be caused by a viral infection such as the common cold, and is also related to an allergy or intolerance to certain foods such as dairy products, leading to the immune system producing masses of mucous. The Eustachian tube is shorter and straighter in children, making it easier for infections to travel up from the throat. The symptoms, which develop gradually and may initially go unnoticed, include partial deafness, immature speech for the child's age, and ear infections. Symptoms tend to fluctuate and worsen in winter months. The gentle heat radiating from the ear candle along with the slight suction effect may encourage the Eustachian tube to open and close properly. An ear candling treatment once a week for a month is recommended, followed by regular monthly treatments.

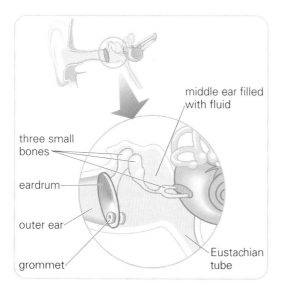

middle ear filled with fluid

three small bones

eardrum

outer ear

grommet

Eustachian tube

Ear grommets

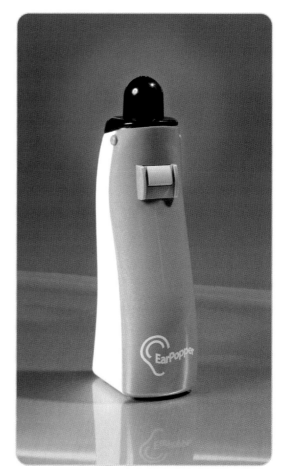

Ear popper

If symptoms persist for several months, myringotomy and grommet insertion is the common operation. Myringotomy is a tiny cut (about 2–3mm) made in the eardrum. The fluid is drained and a grommet (ventilation tube) is often inserted. A grommet is like a tiny pipe that is put across the eardrum. It helps to drain any fluid and allows air to enter the middle ear; hearing improves immediately. Most grommets stay in place for six to twelve months before falling out into the ear canal as the eardrum heals naturally. Ear candling should never be done while grommets are in place.

Adenoids are similar to tonsils but lie at the back of the nose near the opening of the Eustachian tube. If the adenoids are unusually large, taking them out may improve drainage of the Eustachian tube.

A new laser method to make a tiny hole in the eardrum and allow drainage is being developed. This has a similar effect to myringotomy and grommet insertion, and may become more widely available if it proves successful. These operations are carried out under a general anaesthetic and are often done in a day, although an overnight stay in hospital is sometimes needed. Dr Anthony Mathews, a consultant osteopathic otologist, has recorded a high success rate in treating glue ear through osteopathy and dietary changes (see Where to go from here, p 102).

A six-year study in the USA sponsored by the National Institute of Health, involving children diagnosed with hearing loss due to glue ear, showed very positive results with a device called the 'ear popper'. The ear popper directs a steady, controlled stream of air into the nose. Swallowing diverts the air into the

Eustachian tube, opening the Eustachian tube, relieving pressure imbalance in the middle ear and allowing any accumulated fluids to drain (see Useful addresses, page 102).

Hay Fever/Allergic rhinitis

This is the inflammation of the mucous membrane lining the nose and throat due to an allergic reaction to specific inhaled allergens. Such allergens include pollen, perfume, animal hairs and dust. It may occur only in spring and summer, in which case it is known as seasonal allergic rhinitis or hay fever, or it may be perennial and occur all year round. Symptoms include an itchy sensation in the nose, frequent sneezing, blocked or runny nose, and itchy, red, watery eyes. Hay fever and allergic rhinitis are more common in people who have other allergic conditions such as asthma. The anti-inflammatory properties of the ingredients in the ear candles can provide relief, and the tiny amounts of beeswax and honey may have a homeopathic effect on the condition. Depending on the severity of the condition, two to three treatments may be needed in the first week, and then once or twice per week in the next two to three weeks.

Headaches

Headaches can have many causes but dehydration, emotional stress, fatigue or muscular tensions in the upper jaw, scalp and neck area are the principal causes of most headaches.

This leads to constriction of the blood vessels in the area (cutting off blood flow), or dilation (allowing too much blood flow). In many cases, simply drinking more water will alleviate a headache. Ear candling accompanied by massage helps regulate blood circulation and reduces stress on the cranial nerves. The muscles in the area are relaxed and the action of the temporomandibular joint can be improved. The frequency of treatment will depend on the severity of the condition.

Hearing difficulties

Hearing difficulties due to compacted earwax can be alleviated due to the effects of the treatment on softening and loosening the earwax, enabling it to fall out naturally. As hardened earwax softens it expands, and this can lead to an apparent worsening of the hearing loss until the wax is expelled. Several treatments may be required to remove compacted earwax, and regular treatments will prevent this problem from occurring. Hearing difficulties are also a feature of glue ear. Anyone suffering from hearing difficulties or hearing loss should be advised to have the cause medically investigated if not known.

Labyrinthitis

Labyrinthitis (otitis interna) is inflammation of the inner ear, causing vertigo, vomiting, loss of balance and deafness. It is usually due to a bacterial or viral infection. For instance, an infection of the middle ear called acute otitis media may lead to labyrinthitis. An infection of the lining around the brain (meningitis) can also lead to labyrinthitis. This condition should be diagnosed and treated by a doctor. However, an ear candling treatment can help alleviate the stress associated with this condition and improve circulation in the area.

Menière's disease

This is a disorder of the inner ear characterised by episodes of deafness, tinnitus and vertigo, which can vary in severity and frequency. It affects about one in a 1,000 people and most commonly begins between the ages of 20 and 50. One ear is commonly affected at first. The other ear also becomes affected at some stage in about four out of ten cases. Symptoms can last for several hours, and between attacks the affected ear may return to normal, but permanent hearing loss and tinnitus may eventually develop. The exact cause is not known but it is linked to a build-up of fluid in the labyrinth or inner ear,

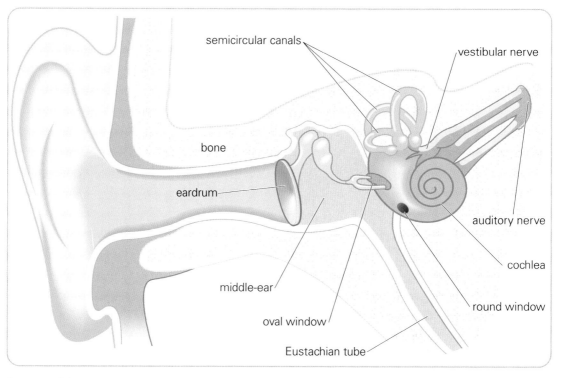

semicircular canals

vestibular nerve

bone

eardrum

auditory nerve

cochlea

middle-ear

round window

oval window

Eustachian tube

Structure of the ear

which may be caused by some fault, where the amount of fluid that you make is more than the amount drained.

Slight abnormalities of the bones around the middle ear as well as inheritance may play some part, as about eight in 100 close relatives of affected people develop Menière's disease, compared to one in a 1,000 of the general population. Other theories include viral infections of the ear, salt imbalance in the labyrinth fluid, diet and a faulty immune system. The build-up of fluid may increase the pressure and cause swelling of the labyrinth, and fluid may leak between different parts of the labyrinth. These effects may cause the inner ear to send abnormal messages to the brain, which causes dizziness and vomiting. The pressure of excess fluid on the hearing cells (which line the labyrinth) is probably why they

do not work so well, and leads to hearing problems. As the pressure eases, the cell function improves and hearing can return to normal. However, repeated bouts of increased pressure may eventually damage the hearing cells, leading to permanent hearing loss. For the sufferer, Menière's disease is a very distressing condition, and an ear candling treatment can help improve local circulation and alleviate the associated stress. There is currently no cure, but treatment can help to ease and prevent symptoms. A low salt diet is usually recommended to reduce the fluid build-up in the inner ear, and avoidance of certain things which seem to trigger the condition (including tobacco, caffeine and alcohol). After-care advice should include information about self-help organisations such as the Menière's Society (see Useful addresses, page 102).

Migraines

Migraines are throbbing, intense and often debilitating headaches, usually occurring on one side of the head and sometimes accompanied by nausea, vomiting and sensitivity to sound, smell or light. They begin slowly and can last for several hours or even days. The cause is due to spasm followed by dilation of blood vessels, and can be triggered by emotional factors such as shock, stress, diet

(common food triggers are citrus fruits, caffeine, chocolate, cheese and red wine) or they can be hereditary. The candles and the massage both improve the blood circulation, and regular treatments can lessen the frequency of attacks. Clients should be advised to keep a diet diary to check if their migraines are triggered by specific foods.

Obstructive sleep apnoea (OSA)

This condition is characterised by repetitive pauses in breathing during sleep due to the obstruction and/or collapse of the upper airway (throat), usually accompanied by a reduction of oxygen in the blood and followed by awakening to breathe. This is called an

apnoea event. Respiratory effort continues during the episodes of apnoea and the body strains to breathe. Symptoms include loud, frequent snoring with episodes of silence that may last from ten seconds to a minute or more. The end of an apnoea episode is often associated with loud snores, gasps, moans, and mumbling.

Not everyone who snores has apnoea and not everyone with apnoea necessarily snores, though most do and this is probably the most obvious indicator. Your bed mate may notice that you periodically stop breathing during your sleep, or gasp for breath. Excessive daytime sleepiness/fatigue is also experienced, as is falling asleep when you do not intend to. This could be almost anytime you are sitting down, such as while watching television, sitting at a desk, and even while driving a car. Sufferers complain of unrefreshing sleep with feelings of grogginess, dullness, morning headaches and severe dryness of the mouth. Body movements often accompany the awakenings at the end of each apnoea episode, and this, together with the loud snoring, will disrupt the bed partner's sleep and often cause her/him to move to a separate bed or room.

OSA is the most common form of sleep apnoea (about four per cent of men and two per cent of women), but there is also a condition called central sleep apnoea (CSA). This is a condition when the brain does not send the right signals to tell you to breathe when you are asleep. In other words the brain 'forgets' to make you breathe. It can also be associated with weakness of the breathing muscles. The assessment for CSA is often more complicated than for OSA, and the treatment has to be carefully matched to the patient's requirements.

There is also a condition called mixed sleep apnoea, that is a combination of both obstructive and central sleep apnoea. Ear candling can help by relieving congestion in the upper airways and improving breathing. Weight loss is also recommended, as sufferers are commonly overweight with poor muscle tone in the neck area.

Patulous Eustachian tube (PET)

This is a condition whereby the Eustachian tube is persistently open, leading to the sufferer being exposed to all the sounds within the head such as yawning, chewing, swallowing as well as the abnormal perception of one's own breath and voice sounds. This condition is more common in females than in males and in adolescents and adults rather than young children. The causes are unknown, and symptoms include a clogged feeling in the ears, which is relieved by lying down for about 20 minutes.

Under normal resting conditions, the Eustachian tube is closed and only opens with

swallowing or auto-inflation, eg holding and blowing the nose. Vertigo and hearing loss can also occur because patulous Eustachian tube allows excessive pressure changes to occur in the middle ear; these pressure changes are then transmitted to the inner ear through ossicular movement. Patients sometimes sniff repetitively to close the Eustachian tube, and this may lead to long-term negative middle ear pressure. Ear candling may provide some relief by improving the action of the Eustachian tube and as the treatment is done with the client lying down, this relieves the condition.

Pressure changes

Changes in air pressure due to flying or diving can lead to a feeling of pain and pressure in the ears as the eardrum bulges towards the area of lower pressure. This is medically known as barotrauma. To keep air pressure inside and outside the eardrum equal, we have natural 'drainage' tubes (the Eustachian tubes) that connect the middle ears to the back of the nose and throat. Our ears always produce small amounts of fluid; this normally drains down the Eustachian tubes, and is usually in such small amounts that we do not even notice it in the throat. The tubes have one-way valves which allow air to escape from the middle ears to the throat; yawning, chewing or swallowing helps open the valves in the other direction so that air (and sometimes fluid) can go into the middle ears. As an aeroplane descends, the air pressure becomes higher nearer the ground and this pushes the eardrum inwards. To relieve this, the pressure inside the middle ear has to rise quickly. If there is any blockage of the Eustachian tube, it stops air entering the middle ear, then the eardrum is stretched and becomes more and more tense from the outside pressure, causing pain.

Common reasons why this might happen are ear infections, throat infections, hay fever or any condition causing extra mucus in the Eustachian tubes. In some people, the Eustachian tube does not drain very well or is too narrow and becomes easily blocked with mucus. Yawning and swallowing will open up the valves and cut down on the pain. Another commonly used technique is the 'Valsalva Manoeuvre' in which you pinch the nose and blow hard against the nose. This forces air into and up the Eustachian tube to equalise the pressure behind the eardrum. A popping sensation should be felt in the ear as the eardrum returns to its correct position. As soon as the plane starts to descend and a change in pressure is sensed, this should be done and repeated every few seconds until landing whenever the pressure drop sensation is felt. When diving, the increased pressure of the descent also puts pressure on the eardrum. The warmth of the candle may help the Eustachian tube to function properly and help the eardrum regain its correct tension due to pressure changes and expansion in the area. A treatment up to 48 hours before and/or after flying or diving is recommended.

Sinus problems

Sinus problems are very common and can be quite debilitating. The sinuses are air-filled cavities around the nose and eyes, lined with mucous-producing cells. Mucous passes continuously through narrow channels leading from the sinuses to the nasal cavity. These passages can become blocked, leading to a build-up of mucous and inflammation of the sinuses. The most common cause is a viral infection such as the common cold. Sinusitis may be acute (developing and clearing rapidly) or chronic (long term). Symptoms include headache, feelings of congestion, pain and tenderness in the face that tends to worsen on bending down. Sinusitis can be relieved by the warming action of the ear candles when combined with massage of specific sinus release points on the face. In the first few days of acute sinusitis, daily treatments can be given. Monthly treatments help to prevent severity and frequency of attacks. For chronic sinusitis, treat weekly for the first month and then fortnightly for two to three months. A reduction in dairy products is recommended to reduce the amount of mucous in the body.

casestudy

Practitioner Gabriele treated Diane, aged 61, for sinus problems. Gabriele writes:

'Diane presented with long standing blocked sinuses, which are particularly bad in cold weather. Her breathing is shallow and through the mouth and she often suffers from colds. She had her first ever Hopi ear candle treatment with me last week and responded extremely well to the treatment. I have recommended a course of treatments for her.'

Diane writes: 'I really enjoyed my first treatment and have definitely benefited from it. I suffer from blocked sinuses and was particularly bad last week – in fact, since the cold weather arrived, I was waking up several times during the night, feeling particularly blocked. At the beginning of the treatment my breathing was quite shallow, but I was soon breathing more deeply. I found the treatment very comfortable, the smell of the candles was lovely, and the massage was great! I have slept really well since then, without waking up as I usually do, and I am breathing more deeply all the time. I think the treatment is still working and I am looking forward to my next treatment. The ear candles have definitely started to clear my blocked sinuses and I am really pleased that I can look forward to normal breathing instead of snuffling so much!'

Snoring

Snoring is defined as a coarse sound made by vibrations of the soft palate and other tissue in the mouth, nose and throat (upper airway). It is caused by turbulence inside the airway during inhalation. The turbulence is caused by a partial blockage, that may be located anywhere from the tip of the nose to the vocal chords. It is often due to congestion of the upper respiratory airways, or being overweight with loss of muscle tone and fatty deposits around the neck area. The restriction may occur only during sleep, or it may persist all the time and be worse when we are asleep. This is because our muscle tone is reduced during sleep and there may be insufficient muscle tone to prevent the airway tissue vibrating. During waking hours muscle tone keeps the airway in good shape, which is why we do not snore when awake. The loudest snore ever recorded was 69 decibels, almost as loud as a pneumatic drill at 70–90 decibels.

Anything that can improve breathing and prevent having to breathe through the mouth with constant vibration of the soft palate can help alleviate snoring. Ear candling can be very successful in some cases as it can help to decongest the upper respiratory airway and improve breathing. The yoga exercise of alternate nostril breathing is excellent and costs nothing. Avoidance of dairy products, which lead to excess mucous, is recommended. Essential oils, such as eucalyptus and pine, vaporised in the bedroom help to open up the airways and improve breathing.

casestudy

Practitioner Lucretia treated Katherine, aged 28, for excessive snoring. Lucretia writes:

'Katherine, works as a PA in busy London office and lives with her partner of three years. She suffers from both work-related and emotional stress that results in sleep problems and low levels of energy. She suffers from frequent migraines, chronic sinus congestion and complains of excessive snoring.

'Katherine's first three treatments were on a weekly basis. Following the first treatment, Katherine reported that on waking in the morning there was residue of wax on her pillow. She also reported feeling very relaxed and rested, having enjoyed a good night's sleep. Katherine found the treatments relaxing and enjoyable, and by the third treatment she felt her airways to be clearer and her breathing easier. Due to pressure of work, the fourth treatment took place after a gap of three weeks. She presented with congested sinuses and pain in her right ear. After the treatment there were significant deposits of wax in the expired candle used in the right ear. The ear pain had significantly decreased, the sinuses felt clear and breathing easier. After treatment five, Katherine reported that the snoring had significantly improved, ie it was less frequent and less vocal. The migraines had reduced in severity and frequency, she felt generally more energised and less stressed. Katherine is delighted with the results of the treatments and continues to have treatments on a regular basis.'

Sore throat (pharyngitis)

A sore throat and pain on swallowing can result from laryngitis, tonsillitis, colds or flu. Bacterial or viral infection or strain on the voice from shouting or overuse can lead to inflammation. As the throat and ear are connected by the Eustachian tube, infection can travel easily from one to the other. Provided the client is not suffering from a contagious disorder such as influenza, the anti-inflammatory ingredients of the ear candles, the clearing of the airways and the increased circulation can help alleviate some of the symptoms and raise the level of the immune system. Clients should be encouraged to rest the voice until the throat returns to normal. Breathing through the nose should be encouraged to prevent the throat from becoming too dry.

Stress

Stress affects people of all ages, and in the long term it can have many negative effects on both physical and mental health. One of the most pleasant functions of an ear candling treatment is relaxation, which calms and soothes the nervous system; people often fall asleep during the treatment. In many cases, ear candling results in improved sleeping patterns and a reduction of hyperactivity in children. German psychotherapists regularly use ear candles to calm disturbed patients before a therapy session starts. Much evidence exists to show the beneficial effect of relaxing experiences on the whole body.

Swimmer's ear

Swimmer's ear is another kind of earache, experienced frequently in summer. This is a bit of a misnomer, since it can happen without swimming, but it is most commonly seen in people who swim often. Swimmer's ear is a bacterial infection of the ear canal, rather than the eardrum and middle ear. The actual infection is usually a boil on the skin within the canal. This can be in the canal's outer part, whose skin is much like that on the rest of your body, or in the inner 'membranous' part which is much thinner skin and sometimes more likely to be infected if it is irritated. If water sits in the canal for very long, it mixes with the earwax. Bacteria start to grow in the mixture, and the wet skin is easier than dry skin for bacteria to penetrate. With a swimmer's ear, it is important to keep the canal as dry as possible until the infection is gone. Those who are regularly affected should use swimmer's earplugs. Ear candling can help by drying out the ear canal but should NOT be carried out if there is current soreness or infection, as it would be very uncomfortable for the client.

casestudy

Practitioner Rosi carried out an ear candling treatment on her mother, aged 60. She writes:

'My mother's ears felt completely blocked after a swim in the sea. She could not hear very well, so I gave her an ear candling treatment and she had immediate relief. As soon as I had finished, she could hear more clearly and was very happy with the quick result.'

Temporomandibular joint (TMJ) syndrome

This condition affects the hinge joint connecting the temporal bone (which houses the ear) to the mandible or lower jaw. Symptoms include dull pain around the ear, tenderness of the jaw muscles, clicking or popping sounds when opening or closing the mouth, headache, tooth sensitivity and abnormal wearing of the teeth. Causes include improperly aligned teeth, clenching or grinding the teeth, dislocation of the joint due to a severe blow or aggressive dental surgery, or arthritis of the joint. Treatment includes heat or ice application, adjusting or reshaping the teeth, use of a gum shield at night to prevent grinding of the teeth, or surgery. Since one of the functions of the temporomandibular joint is to move earwax away from the eardrum, any dysfunction of this joint can lead to a build-up of earwax causing hearing difficulties. The gentle warmth from the candle along with massage of the area can provide relief from the

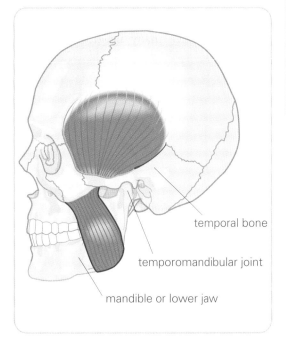

temporal bone

temporomandibular joint

mandible or lower jaw

Temporomandibular joint

symptoms, but the cause should be medically investigated. Cranial osteopathy can be successful in helping to gently realign the joint.

Tinnitus

Tinnitus is a constant or intermittent hissing, buzzing or ringing noise in the ear in the absence of an external sound source. It is a common condition and can occur at any age. Most people have an occasional episode of buzzing tinnitus after going to a loud concert, but this is usually temporary and soon goes. However, about one in 100 people have tinnitus which persists most of the time and affects their quality of life. It may arise from a disorder of the Eustachian tube, or may be due to excessive wax in the ear. It may also be due to chronic muscle tension in the head and neck, leading to disrupted blood flow in these areas. Tinnitus is also a common feature of Menière's disease, which is accompanied by gradually increasing deafness. Irritation of the auditory nerve may follow large doses of certain drugs such as aspirin or quinine and lead to tinnitus.

Whatever the reason, many sufferers who have tried ear candling have reported an improvement in their condition. The pleasant sounds from the burning candle distract from the noises within the ear, while the warmth and the massage both stimulate the blood circulation and relax the muscles of the head and neck. The herb ginkgo biloba has a track record of helping to relieve tinnitus, probably due to its ability to relax the arterial walls, increasing blood flow especially in the cranial area. Some doctors in Germany have reported success in treating patients with a mixture of ginkgo biloba to improve vascularisation, and Hypericum per-foratum to improve the mood. Information on this study can be obtained from Biosun. However, as these herbs can interfere with the action of certain drugs, clients should be advised against self-administration without consulting a medical professional. After-care advice can include information about self-help organisations such as the British Tinnitus Association (see Useful Addresses in the Where to Go from Here section).

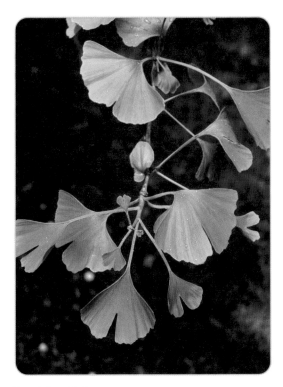

The ginkgo biloba tree

Subtle energy

The blocking of the body's subtle energy creates disorder on a physical, emotional and mental level. Ear candling treatments can promote the release of energy blocks and the flow of subtle energy to facilitate healing. See Chapter 3 for more information.

FAQs

Can I use cotton buds to remove impacted earwax?

Never push cotton buds, fingers or anything else into your ears, as you will push any wax there is onto your eardrum. This could cause pain, infection and deafness. Ask your doctor to check your ears if you think wax has built up.

Do ear candles cure ear diseases?

Although ear candling can alleviate some of the symptoms of ear disease, it is not a cure for these diseases. We recommend that you ask for and follow your doctor's advice concerning any diseases of the ear, and check the contraindications for ear candling to ensure that it is safe to have the treatment.

Does ear candling hurt?

Ear candling carried out by someone who is properly trained and using good quality ear candles will never hurt. The consultation will check for any contraindications such as inflammation in the ear canal, which would make a treatment unpleasant. Most people experience gentle warmth in the ear canal, which has a soothing relaxing effect. There is a slight crackling sound as the candle burns, which most people find very pleasant.

contra-indications

ontraindications are signs or symptoms of presenting conditions that indicate a treatment should not be carried out, or that certain areas should be avoided. 'Contra' means against; 'indication' is a sign. Signs are things that a therapist may notice about a client, such as a scar on the face, whereas symptoms are things that client complains of, or will complain of if appropriate questions are put to them. Contraindications should be checked thoroughly in the initial consultation, and rechecked each time that a client presents for treatment. From a safety viewpoint, if a client presents with a contagious disorder, this can be passed on to the therapist and to other clients, and the condition may be worsened by treatment. Any therapist suffering from a contagious disorder should not carry out treatments.

From a comfort viewpoint, if the client is experiencing pain, the treatment may be counter-productive as they may be too distracted to relax and enjoy the benefits of the treatment. Most importantly, if a client suffers any harm as a result of the

therapist's negligence, it reflects badly on their professionalism and may lead to legal action being taken against them. Therapists should ensure that they have adequate insurance to practise ear candling. Insurance companies require a copy of the training certificate obtained for practice of this therapy and some companies make an extra charge to cover ear candling.

- Some contraindications are total, meaning that the treatment should not be carried out until the condition has completely cleared.

- Others are local contraindications, meaning that the treatment may be carried out but that certain areas should be avoided.

Other presenting conditions may be treated with written advice from the client's medical practitioner. If this advice cannot be obtained, clients must indemnify their condition in writing prior to treatment. This means that they specify their medical condition on the consultation form, agree that all aspects of the

CLIENT CONSULTATION FORM

Name: _____   Date: _____

Address: _____   Client No. _____

_____   Referred by: _____

_____

Email: _____

Telephone: _____   Mobile: _____

D.O.B. _____   U-16 consent form required?

(Ensure consent signed) Y ╪ N

Presenting Condition

(Tick all that apply)

Sinus/rhinitis

Headaches/migraines

Earaches

Tinnitus

Glue ear

Excess/compacted wax

Catarrh

Hay fever

Colds

Sore throats

Snoring

Pressure problems

Meniére's Disease

Other (note below)

Contraindications/Precautions

Perforated ear drums

Ear grommets or tubes

Cochlear implant

Infectious diseases or disorders

Eczema/dermatitis/infections in outer ear

Acute/infectious diseases

High temperature/fever/heavy cold

Recent head or neck injuries

Under influence of alcohol or drugs

High/low blood pressure

Toothache/dental work

Oil in ear

Allergies to ear candle ingredients

Recent operations/scar tissue

Cysts/lumps

Serious medical coditions (specify below)

Other (specify below)

Notes

A sample consultation form

treatment have been fully explained to them and they agree to have the treatment. However it is important that a therapist knows when treatment should definitely not be given and that they do not treat in these cases, even if the client wishes the treatment to go ahead.

When liaising with a client's GP, it is important to be aware that the GP's insurance may not cover them to give their consent to complementary therapy treatments. Therapists should make it clear that they are seeking advice about the suitability of the proposed treatment, and should include literature on ear candling including its methodology, benefits, contraindications and effects. A doctor cannot be expected to give advice about a comple-mentary therapy treatment if they have no knowledge of how it works. This information can take the form of a leaflet, which the therapist uses to advertise their treatments.

Some conditions require additional caution when treating. Outlined below are contraindications and precautions for ear candling and massage, and these should be included in the client's pre-treatment questionnaire. We have included a sample questionnaire for you (opposite), but if you practise several therapies, you may prefer to incorporate this into your own consultation form.

If you are performing solely ear candling (without massage), then the following principles apply.

Conditions that are contraindicated to ear candling

Perforated eardrum

A perforated eardrum (hole in the ear) occurs when the eardrum is damaged following illness or injury. This could occur when a person is subjected to a loud explosion (such as a bomb blast), or when infection in the middle ear causes an accumulation of excessive fluid.

During a treatment, the warm vapours circulate around the ear canal and eardrum. Where the eardrum is perforated, there is a risk that some of the vapour residue or earwax could be deposited in the middle ear. Secondly, the treatment causes the eardrum to vibrate so it needs to heal before treatment can take place.

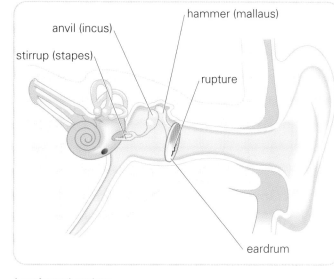

A perforated eardrum

51

Ear grommets or tubes

Devices such as grommets or tubes are placed in the eardrum to facilitate the drainage of excessive fluid from the middle ear following infection. Such devices make a hole in the eardrum. Once the device has been removed or naturally expelled from the ear, it is advisable to wait six months before treatment, to ensure that the eardrum has fully healed.

Eczema or dermatitis in the outer ear

Eczema or dermatitis can sometimes affect the outer ear. It can be extremely itchy and sufferers often scratch their ears during sleep, causing soreness and inflammation. Due to the increased sensitivity, a treatment would feel uncomfortable and cause further irritation to the area.

Cochlear implant

If the client has a cochlear implant – a type of hearing aid – the treatment could interfere with the function of the device and would feel uncomfortable. It is a small electronic device, part of which is implanted in the cochlea and part worn externally. If a client has an external hearing aid only, this should be removed before treatment.

Current or recent infection to the outer ear

Where there is current or recent infection (eg boils) in the outer ear, the ear would be sore and there would be increased sensitivity to the heat and vapours generated during treatment. If infection is in the middle or inner ear, then the treatment should have a beneficial effect. If the client is unsure where the infection is, they should check with their doctor before treatment.

Under the influence of alcohol or drugs

Where a client is under the influence of alcohol or 'recreational' drugs (such as cannabis), a treatment should not take place as it would increase blood flow to the head and may cause dizziness, nausea or irrational behaviour.

Acute infectious diseases

Diseases or infections such as flu, mumps, measles, tuberculosis and chicken pox are contraindicated, as they are highly contagious.

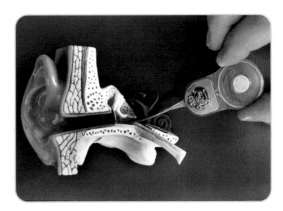

A cochlear implant

High temperature/fever/ heavy cold

If the client is currently unwell with a high temperature/fever, treatment should not take place. This includes if the client has a cold and is sneezing, or has another disease of the respiratory tract where frequent coughing occurs. The infection could be transmitted to the therapist and the client will not be able to enjoy the benefits of the treatment.

Diarrhoea and vomiting

The client will be too distracted to enjoy the benefits of the treatment – the client should investigate the cause of this problem.

Recent head or neck injury

Recent blows to the head with concussion or a recent whiplash injury should not be treated until they have been medically investigated. Such injuries can sometimes dislocate the tiny bones in the middle ear and clients should have this investigated if any hearing loss occurs as a result of the injury.

Skin or scalp infections

Some contagious skin infections such as impetigo, scabies, conjunctivitis, folliculitis, pediculosis capitis (head lice) and tinea capitis (scalp ringworm) are totally contra-indicated to both ear candling and massage as they could be passed on to the therapist and other clients. However some skin infections such as herpes simplex (cold sores) are local contraindications. In this case, avoid the area affected.

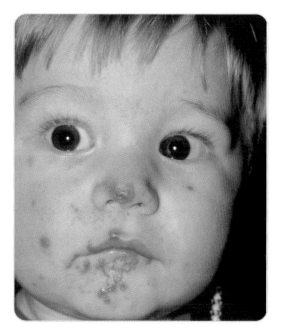

Impetigo

Conditions that require caution when ear candling

Oil placed in the ear

A client may have placed warm oil in the ear to facilitate the removal of earwax. The heat generated by the treatment could make the oil in the ear become very hot, and the vapours could get 'stuck' in the oil, causing residue to accumulate in the ear. A treatment can be given 48 hours after oil has been used.

Allergies

If the client has an allergy or intolerance to any of the constituents of the candles, then a treatment could cause an allergic reaction and discomfort to the client. The ingredients are present in such small amounts that this is rarely a problem but, as a precaution, it is advisable to use a candle brand that does not have the allergen present.

Pregnancy

Pregnancy is not strictly a contraindication to ear candling. Clients may sometimes be more sensitive to smells during pregnancy and prefer a 'basic' candle with no added ingredients.

Sage, which is often one of the ingredients in ear candles, is contraindicated during pregnancy. However, as the amount used in the candles is small, candle manufacturers do not advise pregnancy as a contraindication. Ensure that the client is comfortable and be aware that lying supine or on the right side can put pressure on the inferior vena cava, a large vein that carries de-oxygenated blood from the lower half of the body into the heart.

An on-site massage chair may be more appropriate for a heavily pregnant client.

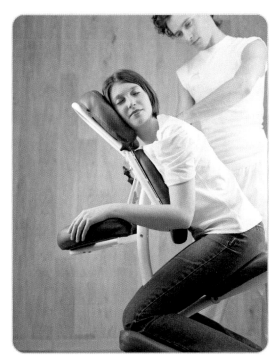

An on-site massage chair

Low blood pressure

Be aware that clients suffering from low blood pressure may experience dizziness when sitting or standing up after treatment, so they should be carefully assisted.

Toothache

If the client is experiencing pain due to toothache or dental work, the treatment may be too uncomfortable for them.

Conditions that may require medical advice before ear candling

Serious medical conditions

If the client has any serious medical conditions, such as cancer, diabetes, thrombosis or heart conditions, they should seek their doctor's advice before a treatment takes place. If a GP or another complementary practitioner has referred the client, keep them informed of the progress. Clients using regular medication (eg for diabetes) should have their necessary medication with them in case of emergency.

High blood pressure

Clients with very high blood pressure are susceptible to the formation of blood clots and the effects of prescribed medication can lead to them feeling dizzy and light-headed after treatment. As massage is said to lower the blood pressure, their medical practitioner should be consulted before treatment so that their medication dose can be monitored and altered by the medical practitioner if necessary.

Epilepsy

Caution is required due to the complexity of this condition and medical advice is recommended. Some smells can trigger epileptic attacks, so bear this in mind when using ear candles or massage oils with strong smells.

Disorders of the nervous system

Clients with disorders of the nervous system such as multiple sclerosis, Parkinson's disease, cerebral palsy, trigeminal neuralgia should consult with their medical practitioner before having a treatment. Gentle massage may help

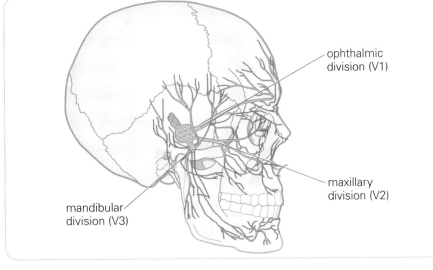

ophthalmic
division (V1)

maxillary
division (V2)

mandibular
division (V3)

Trigeminal nerve distribution

to reduce spasms associated with disorders of the nervous system. Extra care should be taken to ensure the comfort of the client during the treatment, and shorter treatments may be more appropriate.

If you are also performing a massage of the scalp, face, neck and ears, then the following apply IN ADDITION to those listed for ear candling. Bear in mind that the massage is of a very soothing and gentle nature and does not stimulate the cardiovascular system in the way that a full body massage would.

Conditions that require caution when massaging

Recent operations/scar tissue

Depending on the site and the nature of the operation, it may be a total or local contra-indication, or may require medical approval. Do not massage until the tissue is fully healed and can withstand pressure. After that, massage can help to break down adhesions. Some guidelines suggest that scar tissue following a major operation can be massaged after two years and small scars following minor cuts and wounds after six months. In many cases massage can be done sooner depending on the speed of the healing process.

Skin disorders

Some skin disorders such as weeping eczema, dermatitis or psoriasis on the area to be massaged should be treated as local contra-indications, as the area may be raw, sore and prone to infection. Massaging the area could cause infection to spread.

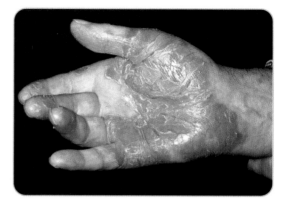
Psoriasis

Undiagnosed lumps, bumps and swellings

Cysts are common in the scalp and can sometimes be painful or sensitive to touch. Mostly they are sebaceous cysts. A treatment is not totally contraindicated but the area of the cyst should be avoided and the client should have any lumps, bumps or swellings medically investigated if they have not already done so.

Bruising, open cuts or abrasions, sunburn

These are usually local contraindications and the area should be avoided during treatment. The cause of any bruising should be checked with the client as this could indicate an underlying medical condition.

Doubts

If you have any doubts about the suitability of a client for treatment, SEEK PROFESSIONAL ADVICE and DO NOT TREAT until you feel that it is safe to do so.

Side effects

Side effects of this gentle treatment are usually positive rather than negative, and the client consultation should alert you to any possible reactions. The whole treatment, particularly the massage, encourages the systems of the body to function more efficiently. This can result in speeding up waste removal from the body through the cardiovascular and lymphatic systems. Therefore there are some possible side effects that your clients may be aware of for a few days following the treatment, which may or may not include the following:

- increase in urination due to stimulation of the circulation
- increased thirst, due to increased urination
- increase or other changes in bowel movements due to stimulation of the parasympathetic nervous system and more efficient elimination of waste
- headaches or light-headedness due to increased circulation and elimination of toxins – drinking water after a treatment usually prevents headaches occurring

- increase in mucous from nasal passages as sinuses are draining following facial massage
- change in sleep pattern, usually improved
- Increase in appetite, due to increase in metabolic rate
- increase in sensitivity in terms of emotions
- feeling of tiredness, often leading to feeling revitalised
- relief of stress and tension in muscles and joints
- feeling of fullness in the ears as wax is hydrated and expands following treatment
- hearing may be temporarily impaired (in the same way as it is following the use of oil or eardrops that hydrate impacted earwax). More treatments may be required to loosen the wax before it is expelled naturally.

FAQs

How would I know if a client had a perforated eardrum?

A perforated eardrum is a hole or rupture in the eardrum, which separates the ear canal and the middle ear. It is often accompanied by decreased hearing and occasional discharge. Pain is usually not persistent. The causes of perforated eardrum are usually trauma or infection, so if the above symptoms are present, you would ask about recent ear infections, strong blows to the ear, head injuries, exposure to loud sounds such as an explosion and use of cotton buds or other implements in the ear. Do not treat, and refer the client to their doctor if you suspect a perforated eardrum. If you have been trained and insured to use an otoscope, you can examine the eardrum.

If my client is in a wheelchair or is otherwise unable to lie on a massage couch, can I still perform the treatment?

You can perform the treatment as long as the client can comfortably tilt their head and rest it on a support such as one or more cushions. The ear candle should be inserted as vertically as possible for optimal results. Some therapists carry out the treatment quite successfully on a reflexology or on-site massage chair, and this may be more suitable for heavily pregnant clients. The massage may be omitted in this case and the treatment can be done with ear cones, which have a shorter burning time.

How would I know if my client were having an allergic reaction to the ingredients of the ear candle, and what would I do?

Very rarely, allergic reactions are reported. This takes the form of spontaneous itching and if it occurs, the treatment should be stopped. Some oil (such as olive, jojoba or safflower) can be applied to soothe the area. Do not drop the oil into the ear but massage lightly around the outer opening of the ear canal.

an ear candling treatment

Procedure

Preparation

- Prepare the room in advance. A clean, fresh environment can encourage the client to relax more readily, and it enhances the effects of the treatment. Use a room that is quiet with soft lighting and free from draughts (or powerful fans in summer), as this may cause the candle to be extinguished or ash to blow onto the client.

- Check the location of smoke alarms as some ear candles may trigger these to go off during the treatment. However, this is rarely a problem with good quality beeswax ear candles.

- When doing the ear candling, music is not necessary as it can overload the senses and distract from the pleasant sounds of the candle burning. Some clients enjoy listening to relaxing music while the massage is being carried out, while others prefer silence.

- Allow adequate time for the treatment to take place. Taking into account the pre-treatment consultation, the ear candling, the massage and after-care advice, a full treatment will take approximately 45 minutes.

The therapist

- For safety purposes, the treatment should not be self-administered. The treatment is very relaxing and it is possible to fall asleep during a treatment.

- The therapist's appearance should be clean, tidy and professional.

- Nails should be short so they do not interfere with the massage.

- Bracelets and watches should be removed.

- Long hair should be tied back for safety and hygiene purposes.

Equipment

Have everything ready for the treatment before the client arrives. Items needed for the treatment should be within easy reach of the therapist on a small table or trolley. Here is a list of the items you will require:

- massage couch set up with couch cover, towels, blankets, pillow etc. When purchasing a couch, ensure that you can sit comfortably with your knees underneath

- chair, which should be a comfortable height so that elbows can rest on the couch by the client's head; a height-adjustable chair or stool is best

- pair of ear candles or cones

- lighter, matches or a small lighted candle nearby from which to light the ear candles

- water to extinguish the ear candles after use

- cloth with a hole for the ear to protect the client's face/head. (For suppliers see Useful Addresses in the Where to Go from Here section)

- cotton buds to gently wipe away any powder residue that can adhere to the tiny hairs at the entrance of the ear canal

- tissues

- consultation form and pen

- clock to time how long each candle takes to burn down to the marker line

- bolster to place under client's knees (for the massage)

- drinking water and glass

- container for client's jewellery or valuables

- massage oil (if required).

When the client arrives

- Complete the client consultation form, checking for any contraindications. A sample form has been included in Chapter 5.

- For children under 16, a parent or guardian must be present throughout the treatment and sign the under-16 consent form. Children can be treated from the age of 3, after assessing their suitability in terms of excitability and ability to lie still for the duration of a treatment. See safety precaution guidelines on page 70.

- Explain the treatment to the client, including the fact that they do not have to undress, and assure them that they will not be burned or harmed in any way. Advise the client not to chat through the treatment and tell them that it is important to inform you if they experience discomfort at any time during the treatment. Tell them what to expect during the treatment:

  - a pleasant crackling sound will be heard

  - gentle heat will be experienced around the ear

  - a 'popping' sensation may be experienced.

- The client removes shoes, tight belts or ties and any heavy over-garments. Glasses, external hearing aids, necklaces/neck chains, earrings and hair accessories should be removed and set aside. Some types of contact lenses may need to be removed.

- Make a note of which candle is being used on the right and left side of the client. You can do this by marking 'L' for left and 'R' for right just below the safety marker line on each candle.

CONSENT FOR CHILDREN UNDER 16 YEARS

Name: _____

Address: _____

_____

_____

_____

Telephone: _____

I, _____ (name of parent/guardian), have been advised that according to law I should consult a doctor concerning the health of my child.

After taking this advice I consent to _____ (name of child) having an Ear Candle treatment and accept full responsibility for the treatment/course of treatments being carried out.

Signature of parent/guardian _____

Date _____

A sample under-16 consent form

୬ The therapist washes his/her hands and the client lies on their side on the couch. As the therapist usually starts treatment on the side where the client considers their problem to be most severe, that side should be uppermost.

୬ Ensure the client is warm and comfortable by covering them with a blanket, providing adequate pillow support for their head and a pillow or bolster to support their arms when lying on the side. Over the hair and forehead, place a cloth in which a small hole has been cut to allow the ear to be seen. This ensures that no hair can reach the flame and makes the client feel reassured that they will be protected.

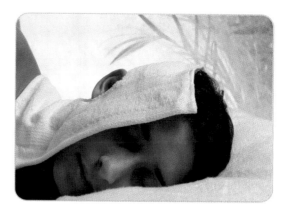

A client ready for treatment

୬ Visually inspect the outer part of the ear to ensure that there is no inflamed skin that the client may have forgotten to disclose in the consultation.

61

Position of the candle

🜆 Before lighting the candle, allow the client to experience what it feels like to have it inserted by holding it in position just inside the auditory canal. It should be as vertical as possible and should not feel uncomfortable or painful. The candle should NEVER be pushed down into the ear canal, but is gently twisted and the ear lobe gently pulled back to obtain a good seal.

🜆 The candle is then withdrawn and lit horizontally away from the client. For Biosun candles, light away from the filter at the unlabelled end. For ear cones, light the non-pointed end. For other ear candles, follow the manufacturer's instructions.

🜆 The non-burning end is then inserted in the client's ear as above. Cylindrical candles such as those made by Biosun

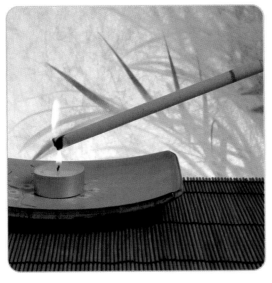

Lighting a candle

have a straight seam and this should point towards the client's face so that when it burns down, any ash (which is not normally hot) will fall away from the client's face (the ash tends to fall backwards from the seam). A light turning movement should be applied so that the ear candle is sealed, and this seal can be assisted with a gentle pull of the client's ear lobe.

🜆 Make a note of what time the lit candle is placed into the ear.

🜆 If the candle is inserted properly, no mist should emerge from the base of the lighted ear candle while it is in the ear. If mist is seen coming from the base of the candle, gently reposition it until this stops occurring. A simple twisting movement usually achieves this. This mist or white smoke is the result of the vapourised ingredients, which are drawn down inside the hollow tube of the ear candle to circulate in the outer ear canal.

How to hold the candle

🜆 The candle should be secured with the first two fingers of one hand, with the remaining fingers resting on the client. The other hand can be gently placed on the client's head or rested nearby on the pillow. When working on the right ear, it is best to hold the candle with the right hand, and vice versa when working on the left ear, so that you are not covering the client's face with your arm.

🜆 Care should be taken not to lean on the client or place undue pressure on the head during treatment.

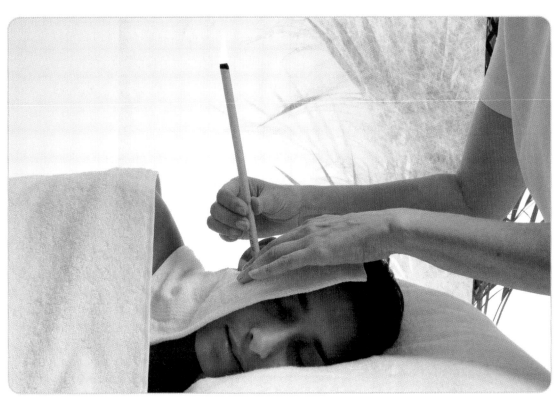

Placing the lighted ear candle in position

What the client experiences

- If the candle is securely in place, the client will experience gentle heat from the vapours, which are drawn down inside the hollow tube of the ear candle. They will also experience a pleasant crackling or sizzling sound as the ingredients impregnated in the fabric of the ear candle burn to create these vapours. The sound increases as the ear candle burns down, and is more easily heard when compacted earwax or sensorineural problems have not affected the hearing.

- They may experience a feeling of pressure being released in the ears or sinuses, or a popping sound as the Eustachian tube opens.

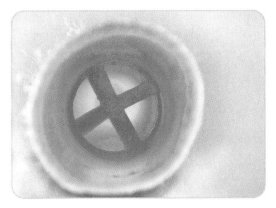

Close-up view of the filter in a Biosun ear candle

63

In good quality ear candles made with beeswax, there should be little or no black smoke coming up from the top of the candle. However, if smoke is present, this may be an indicator of problems or blockages in the ear, nose or throat area, and the client consultation and analysis of the ear candle residue will usually confirm this.

Ear candles or cones with a filter prevent large particles of wax or other residue entering the ear.

Removing the candle from the ear

If the client experiences any discomfort during the treatment, eg extreme sensitivity to the heat, then the candle should be immediately removed.

For Biosun candles, once the candle has burnt down to approximately 1 cm above the marker line (about two-thirds of its length) and NO FURTHER, it should be removed carefully and the flame

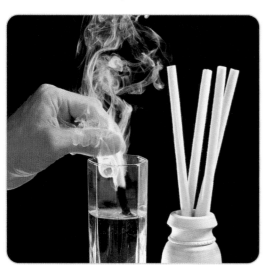

An ear candle being extinguished

extinguished in a glass of water. Do not completely immerse the candle in the water. For other candles or ear cones, follow the manufacturer's instructions.

Put the used candle to one side so the residue can be checked after treatment.

After the candle is removed

Make a note of how long the candle took to burn down.

Check for any herbal residue from the candle that may be deposited in the client's outer ear – this can be gently removed. It is quite common for a small amount of the herbal residue from the ear candle to descend below the filter, but due to the shape of the ear canal and the protection of its entrance by tiny hairs, the residue cannot travel down the ear canal. As we are only touching the edge of the outer ear, a good quality cotton bud may be used. DO NOT PUT/PUSH ANYTHING DOWN THE EAR CANAL.

Ask the client to turn over to the other side, and repeat the treatment in the other ear.

On completion of both ears, the client should rest for 10–15 minutes. During this rest period, the treatment can be enhanced by a soothing massage of the face, neck, ears and scalp; this helps to increase circulation, relax tense muscles, further clear the sinuses and promote relaxation – see Chapter 7 for a suggested massage sequence.

After the treatment

- Assist the client to sit up slowly, help them off the couch, wash your hands and offer them a glass of water.
- Ask how they felt during and after the treatment. Deposits of wax and or powder may accumulate in or around the candle's filter.
- Open the candles and look at this residue as a partial indicator of how frequent treatments should be.

After-treatment advice

Following the treatment it is important to give some simple advice that will enable the client to gain the utmost benefit from the treatment. Here are some suggestions:

- Drink some water after the treatment; this will promote the elimination of toxins and should prevent the occurrence of a post-treatment headache.
- To enjoy the full benefits of the treatment, it is advisable to avoid water sports such as swimming for 24 hours after treatment.

- Very occasionally the ears may feel more sensitive to the environment on the day following treatment. Avoid cold winds and draughts if possible, or place a small amount of cotton wool in the ears (just at the entrance to the ear canal and no further down).
- Never poke at the ears with cotton buds or any other instruments, as you may damage the eardrum.
- Reduce intake of dairy products if you suffer from sinus problems, as these create excess mucous in the body.
- Cut down on caffeinated drinks and alcohol, as these have a diuretic effect on the body.
- Instead increase intake of water, herbal teas or fresh juices to keep all the cells of the body hydrated and assist the process of waste removal.
- Take time out for regular relaxation.
- Have regular treatments to keep the ears and upper respiratory system free of congestion.

Frequency of treatments

The effects of the treatment can continue to work for up to 48 hours after the treatment, eg pressure balancing and removal of earwax, so treatments should be at least two days apart. Following a client's first treatment, a guide to the frequency of further treatments can be determined by:

- purpose of the treatment, ie what the client is aiming to achieve

- severity of conditions presented by the client
- results of the treatment, ie immediate effects and effects over days following the treatment
- analysis of post-treatment residue.

Purpose of the treatment

Why did the client have a treatment?

The therapist should determine what the client is aiming to achieve from the treatment. For example:

- The purpose is to clear compacted earwax – this may clear after one treatment or take two or more treatments.

- The client had a headache following jetlag – this may clear after one treatment.

Severity of conditions

Are the conditions mild, acute or chronic?

The more severe the conditions, the more treatments will be needed. For example:

- A condition such as chronic sinus problems will usually require a minimum of three treatments with a gap of no more than a week between each of these treatments. Maintenance treatments once or twice a month to minimise symptoms should follow this.

- An acute condition, such as a cold, may require two to three treatments per week until symptoms are cleared.

Results of the treatment

What immediate results did the client feel?

The client will usually feel immediate benefit from the treatment, ie relief from presenting conditions. For example:

- A headache may completely clear, sinuses feel less congested or ears feel less blocked.

- Unless symptoms are completely clear, the client could benefit from further treatments.

How did the client feel 48 hours after treatment?

For example:

- Reduced hearing can accompany a symptom of compacted ear wax. Following treatment, hearing may be further reduced temporarily due to the ear wax hydrating and expanding. Hearing should improve after a day or two as the ear wax is naturally expelled.

Analysis of post-treatment residue

After a treatment, the candles can be opened and the residue inside observed. There is much debate among practitioners regarding the analysis of the post-treatment residue, with some claiming that it comes from the clients' ears and others disregarding the residue and basing the results of the treatment on the reactions of the client.

It is very obvious that this residue does not come from the client's ears; in ear candles which contain a filter, the residue is found ABOVE the filter only. This point reinforces the importance of using candles which contain a filter, as otherwise the residue can end up in the clients' ears, one of the main reasons that ear candling has received some negative publicity.

The residue is actually beeswax and powder from the ear candle itself, and can also be found by simply burning an ear candle down

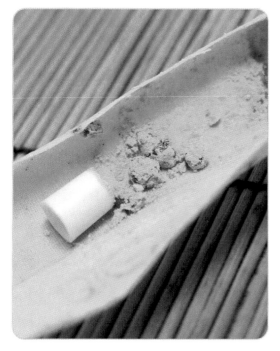

The candle residue remains above the filter

without inserting it into an ear, allowing it to cool and opening it.

From our experience in treating clients over a number of years, and the experience of many other therapists, it has been observed that more wax and powder residue is found with clients whose problems are more severe. Also, more wax and powder residue is generally found on the side where ear, nose or throat problems are more severe, and the candle can take longer to burn on that side. Problems such as compacted earwax may decrease the space for the vapours to circulate, and problems with other parts of the ear and related structures may sap the heat energy from the candle rather than allowing it to be used in burning off the ingredients. The more severe the condition, the more residue is usually present above the filter after treatment.

The amount of this wax and powder residue that accumulates in the candle can be used as an indication of how often the client needs treatments, together with a discussion with the client on the effects of the treatment. Often the results will differ between the two ears, with more residue found on one side than the other.

Below is a guideline to frequency of treatments indicated by candle residue:

Clear results

If the candle has burned cleanly leaving no residue, this may indicate no problems in the ear, nose and throat area. So far in our practice, we have not come across a case where no reside was present after treatment. Due to environmental pollution, particularly in city environments, allergens and mucous-forming foods such as dairy products in the diet, this is very uncommon. Most people experience mild congestion from time to time, often causing no major discomfort. If no residue remains in the candle after treatment, treatments every four to six months would be suggested as a preventative measure, or more frequently if the client enjoys the treatment and finds it an effective way to de-stress.

Small amount of residue

An example of a small amount would be only the yellow powder, which is the herbal residue from the candle. This may indicate a slight problem such as a mild sinus problem or a slight cold, and is quite a common result. Some of the heat energy from the candle may be working to treat the problem, so not as much heat is rising to burn the candle ingredients, which then accumulate above the filter. In this case, four to six weeks is usually recommended until the next treatment, but the client may wish to have more frequent treatments for relaxation purposes.

ear candling in essence

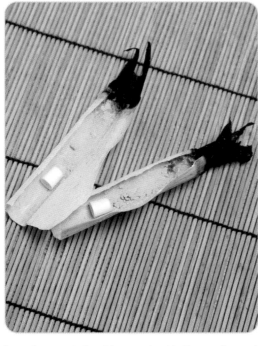

A small amount of residue remained in the candle used on the client's left ear, and a medium amount on the right ear. This client indicated problems on the right side before treatment

Medium amount of residue

An example of this would be a small amount of beeswax and usually some yellow powder. This is often found with more severe problems such as headaches, flu or sinusitis. More heat energy may be working around the eardrum, leaving less to burn off the wax and the herbal ingredients, which remain above the filter. In this case, treatment every two to four weeks is recommended until the condition improves.

Large amount of residue

This would be larger amounts of beeswax and powder and usually indicates more severe problems such as acute or chronic sinus problems, migraines, tinnitus, etc. Most of the heat energy from the candle is probably dissipated around the eardrum, leaving little to burn off the candle ingredients, which remain as wax and powder above the filter. In this case, treatments once or twice a week for three weeks are advised, with monthly treatments recommended as maintenance.

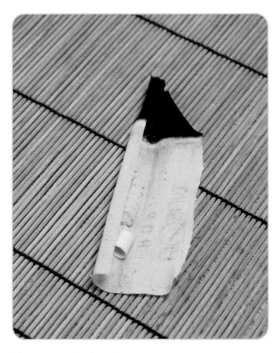

A large amount of residue

FAQs

What is an otoscope, and should I use one in my ear candling treatments?

An otoscope is a medical instrument consisting of a magnifying lens and light. It is used for examining the external ear (the auditory meatus) and the tympanic membrane or eardrum. It is used in conjunction with a speculum, an instrument that holds an opening of the body open so that an examination can be performed. You can obtain a home otoscope from a medical supply store for about £150, but home otoscopes are of dramatically lower quality than the instruments a medical doctor uses, which are far more expensive. You should NOT use this equipment without adequate training and insurance. Information on minimum training requirements can be obtained from the British Society of Audiology, whose contact details can be found in Chapter 9, the useful addresses section.

What can I do if the entrance to the ear canal is very tiny?

Ear cones which have a smaller base are suitable in this case. If using the Biosun candles, you can gently squeeze the base of the candle to make it a bit smaller. However, be careful never to push the base of the candle too far down the ear canal as this will be very uncomfortable and is potentially dangerous. The client should always be told to inform you immediately of any discomfort.

Is it important to show the residue to the client after treatment?

The candle residue is of interest, but placing too much emphasis on its importance can detract from the effectiveness of the treatment. Some clients find it difficult to accept that the residue does not come from the ears. Show it to a client if you consider it

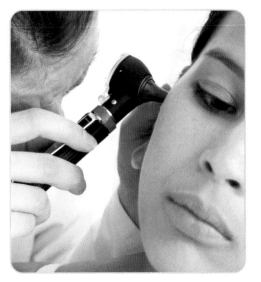

An otoscope

appropriate, eg where there are significant amounts of residue, or where more residue is present in the candle used on the side where more problems exist.

Should I use more than one ear candle on each ear during a treatment?

The effects of the candles are powerful, and it is not necessary to use more than one candle per ear during a treatment. Using more than one candle in each ear could over stimulate the area and make the ears sore.

My three-year-old daughter suffers from earache. Is it a good idea to treat her?

Children as young as three years can be treated as long as they are able to remain still while the ear candle is in place. Ear cones which have a shorter burning time are suitable for young children or half a candle may be used in each ear. The following case study may help to answer this question for you.

casestudy

Practitioner Luma writes:

'I have two daughters, Munia aged five and Rana aged three and a half. Munia is a very energetic happy child and she asked me to do ear candling on her because she saw me do it on her dad, so I have used ear candles on her several times. She loves it and usually lies down on the sofa and becomes very calm and relaxed. I always wanted to use ear candles on Rana, because she suffers from frequent ear infections and a blocked nose, but I felt that perhaps she was too young. However, last week she really wanted me to do it as she had earache in her right ear and her nose was very congested, so I was happy to give it a try. I put her on the sofa, put some cartoons on TV and sat beside her head, holding the ear candle in her ear to show her how it felt. Then I lit the candle and put it in her ear. Rana was very relaxed and we talked quietly and watched the cartoon. When we had finished both ears, I showed her the residue inside the candle. Sure enough, there was a lot of residue from her right ear, which was troubling her. That night she slept really well, her blocked nose cleared and her appetite improved. I have continued to use Hopi ear candles on Rana as a preventative measure because of the cold weather and a lot of children being ill in the nursery. Sometimes I use one full candle on each ear, and sometimes half a candle if she has difficulty lying still. I am amazed at her recovery which once again proved to me how wonderfully ear candling works – not only does it clear the sinuses, but also it helps young children to relax. I suggest that for very young children like Rana it is best to do the treatment when they come home from nursery or in the late afternoon after a snack and when they are tired. You can use nice music or watch a cartoon with them. It really works!'

SAFETY PRECAUTIONS IN THE TREATMENT OF CHILDREN

- Children should not be treated unless they wish to have the treatment and have the ability to lie still and communicate to the parent or therapist how they are feeling before, during and after the treatment.

- A parent or legal guardian should always be present when a child is being treated and consent of the child and parent/guardian should be documented

- A parent or guardian should observe the child for up to 48 hours after treatment and ensure they drink plenty of liquids to help with any detoxifying effects of the treatment.

- We recommend that manufacturers' guidelines be followed in the treatment of children. Biosun and Otosan state that their products can safely be used on children aged 3 upwards. However, some professional organisations recommend that children should be older before being treated (e.g. 7–10 years old). If you are a qualified therapist, check the guidelines of your professional organisation.

- We recommend that only products that have been tested for quality and safety and that conform to medical device directive 93/42/EEC should be used on children.

- Ear Candling is a complementary therapy and should not substitute medical treatment if this appears necessary. In some cases, doctor's advice may be required to ensure there is no medical reason why the treatment should not be carried out.

massage

An ear candling treatment can be enhanced by massage of the face, neck, scalp and ears. This sequence includes effleurage, pressure points, gentle friction and lymphatic drainage, and combined with ear candling, the whole treatment should take around 45 minutes. The massage may be omitted if the client does not wish to have it due to time constraints or personal preference, or if they present with contraindications to massage.

Massage has many benefits to all systems of the body. It stimulates the parasympathetic nervous system, which decreases the heart rate, lowers blood pressure and dilates blood vessels helping them to work more efficiently.

It slows down and deepens respiration, and improves lung capacity by relaxing any tightness in the respiratory muscles. As these systems relax, peristalsis is encouraged as the digestive system begins to work better and more blood flows to the reproductive organs, which receive a reduced blood supply in times of stress.

The psychological effects include a reduction in stress and anxiety, a feeling of wellbeing and enhanced self-esteem, positive body awareness and an improved body image.

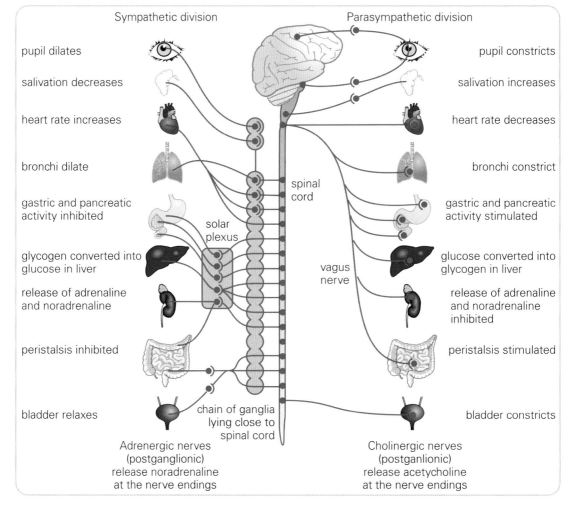

Sympathetic division

pupil dilates

salivation decreases

heart rate increases

bronchi dilate

gastric and pancreatic
activity inhibited

glycogen converted into
glucose in liver

release of adrenaline
and noradrenaline

peristalsis inhibited

bladder relaxes

chain of ganglia
lying close to
spinal cord

Adrenergic nerves
(postganglionic)
release noradrenaline
at the nerve endings

solar
plexus

spinal
cord

Parasympathetic division

pupil constricts

salivation increases

heart rate decreases

bronchi constrict

gastric and pancreatic
activity stimulated

glucose converted into
glycogen in liver

release of adrenaline
and noradrenaline
inhibited

peristalsis stimulated

bladder constricts

vagus
nerve

Cholinergic nerves
(postganlionic)
release acetycholine
at the nerve endings

The two divisions of the autonomic nervous system

Massage techniques

Holding

This is the term used for gently placing the hands over the client's ears and crown of head, and holding each position for five seconds. This lightest of touches is registered by the brain, and this is a soothing way to start and close a massage sequence.

Effleurage

This term derives from 'effleurer', a French word meaning 'to touch lightly'. It is a gentle, sweeping, relaxing stroke, with varying levels of pressure, used at the beginning and end of a massage, to soothe, relax and improve circulation. It prepares the body for massage,

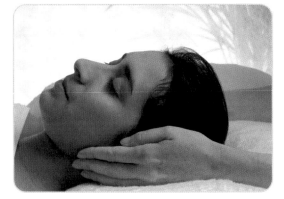

Gently holding the head is very calming

introduces the client to the therapist's touch and warms the area. Effleurage encourages desquamation of skin cells, and increases sebum production, helping to improve the skin's suppleness and resistance to infection. It also encourages vasodilation, bringing oxygen and nutrients to skin cells and speeding up the removal of waste such as lactic acid.

On the face, we do this gentle sweeping movement using both hands. All movements start at the mid-line and move in an outward direction.

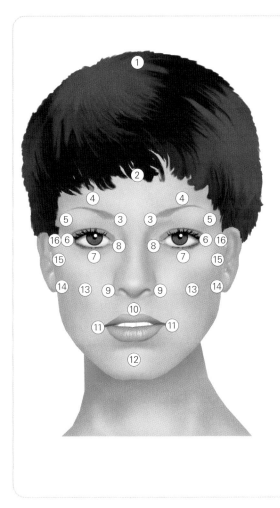

These points are located along meridian lines. As well as activating the energy of that meridian and the organs connected with it, some of these points aid other functions within the body. Make small circles or pump each point gently with your fingers. If you do this regularly you can improve the free flow of qi in your body and improve your health and wellbeing.

Point 1: Governing Vessel 20 – relieves depression and clears the mind

Point 2: Governing Vessel 23 – relieves headaches and migraines; this point also corresponds to the third eye chakra

Point 3: Urinary Bladder 2 – helps facial paralysis, eg Bell's palsy, relieves tired eyes

Point 4: Gall Bladder 14 – alleviates headaches

Point 5: Triple Heater 23 – relieves eye problems, headaches and facial paralysis

Point 6: Gall Bladder 1 – relieves conjunctivitis, migraine, tension headaches

Point 7: Stomach 1 – relieves conjunctivitis, glaucoma, cataracts; brightens eyes

Point 8: Urinary Bladder 1 – relieves conjunctivitis and insomnia

Point 9: Large Intestine 20 – good for any nose problems, facial paralysis, common cold

Point 10: Governing Vessel 26 – good for gum pain or swelling, diminishes hunger so good for weight reduction

Point 11: Stomach 4 – good for facial paralysis

Point 12: Conception Vessel 24 – good for facial paralysis and toothache

Point 13: Stomach 3 – good for facial paralysis, trigeminal neuralgia and nasal obstructions

Point 14: Gall Bladder 2 – stimulates gall bladder meridian and lymph nodes located in the area

Point 15: Small Intestine 19 – good for ear disorders, tinnitus, deafness, stimulates lymph nodes located in the area

Point 16: Triple Heater 21 – stimulates this meridian and lymph nodes located in the area

Facial acupressure points

Pressure points

This is the application of pressure to specific points using the fingers. Applying pressure to these points releases blocked energy, improves circulation, encourages decongestion of the sinuses and stimulates the nerves. Eight of the 14 major acupuncture meridians have points on the face, so it is no surprise that facial acupressure can have such a profound effect on the whole body. Use the diagram on page 73 to apply gentle pressure as indicated.

Friction

The name comes from the Latin word 'fricare' which means to rub down. Friction techniques are used to compress tissue against bone, ie they do not involve sliding across the skin. Friction movements are done either using the whole hand or just the fingers, thumbs, or palm. It is often used for close work on a small area, or on specific areas of tightness such as the temporomandibular joint. If this joint is not working efficiently, it can lead to a build-up of compacted earwax. Friction improves circulation, releases muscular tension in the muscles of mastication such as the masseter muscle, and encourages hair growth when carried out on the scalp. Pressure is varied according to the area being worked, from medium pressure in areas such as the back of neck, to light pressure in areas such as the face. In this sequence, the finger pads of three fingers of each hand are used on large areas (eg forehead and cheeks) and one or two fingers are used on small areas (eg above the mouth). Movements should be circular and gentle over the face, neck and scalp, and four to five circles should be done in each position.

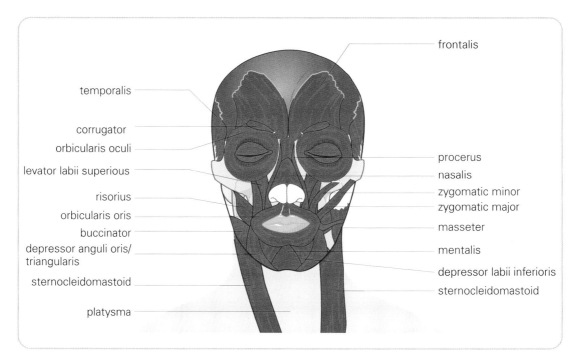

Friction releases tension from the facial muscles

Lymphatic drainage

The lymphatic system is intimately connected with the cardiovascular system. Lymph is a clear, straw-coloured fluid similar to plasma, the fluid part of blood. It starts out as plasma, flowing through the arteries carrying oxygenated blood and nutrients to supply all the cells of the body. Plasma leaks out of the tiny capillaries and into spaces between the cells in the tissues to become tissue fluid. This bathes the cells, providing oxygen and nutrients essential for energy, growth, and renewal, as well as removing bacteria and waste from the cells. Some of the fluid is picked up by the blood capillaries where it becomes plasma again, but excess fluid containing waste molecules that are too large to enter the blood capillaries is drained into lymphatic capillaries which join together to form lymphatic vessels, and the fluid is now called lymph. The lymph flows in a closed network of vessels in a system that is completely separate from the blood circulation.

The lymphatic system has no pump of its own, so to flow efficiently it relies on the movement of nearby muscles, eg when breathing or walking. As muscles contract, they squeeze the lymph along the lymphatic vessels, which have valves to prevent the fluid flowing back. Located at intervals along the lymphatic vessels are oval or bean-shaped organs called lymph nodes containing specialised white blood cells called lymphocytes, which destroy certain bacteria, viruses and other pathogens. These nodes act as filters for the lymph, cleaning it up before it eventually returns to the bloodstream via two lymphatic ducts which empty into the right and left subclavian veins in the neck. At night, when this drainage system slows down, fluid builds up in the tissues. That is why your face can appear puffy first thing in the morning. Lack of physical exercise during the day as well as poor diet, pollution, and shallow breathing can all restrict lymphatic drainage and slow the flow of lymph. If the lymph system gets overloaded you can see the effect in the condition of your skin, such as the appearance of spots, blackheads, and dry patches.

Massaging the face helps to speed up blood and lymph drainage and ensures that the

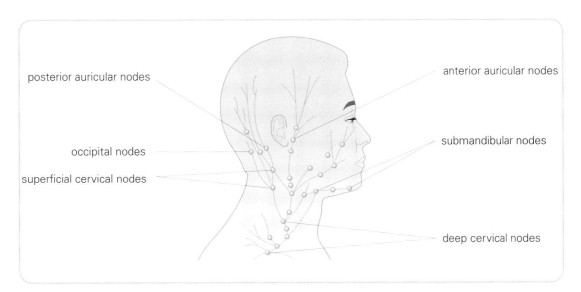

Lymph nodes of the head and neck

ear candling in essence

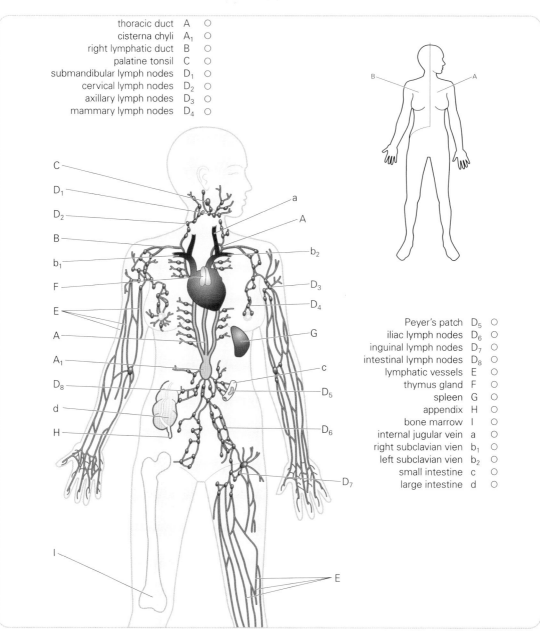

thoracic duct	A	○
cisterna chyli	A_1	○
right lymphatic duct	B	○
palatine tonsil	C	○
submandibular lymph nodes	D_1	○
cervical lymph nodes	D_2	○
axillary lymph nodes	D_3	○
mammary lymph nodes	D_4	○

Peyer's patch	D_5	○
iliac lymph nodes	D_6	○
inguinal lymph nodes	D_7	○
intestinal lymph nodes	D_8	○
lymphatic vessels	E	○
thymus gland	F	○
spleen	G	○
appendix	H	○
bone marrow	I	○
internal jugular vein	a	○
right subclavian vien	b_1	○
left subclavian vien	b_2	○
small intestine	c	○
large intestine	d	○

Lymphatic circulation of the body

vessels are cleansed of waste products that have not been removed naturally. There are important lymph nodes in the armpits, groin and the back of the knees, but many nodes are located near the ears and in the neck, and by stimulating these you will soon see a difference in your face. You will notice that your complexion will start to glow and you will have a more efficient immune system.

As lymphatic vessels are located close to the

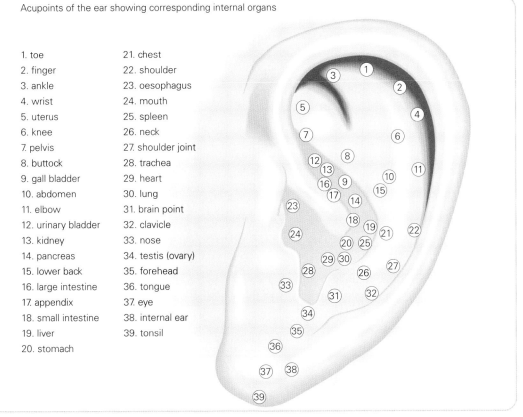

Acupoints of the ear showing corresponding internal organs

1. toe
2. finger
3. ankle
4. wrist
5. uterus
6. knee
7. pelvis
8. buttock
9. gall bladder
10. abdomen
11. elbow
12. urinary bladder
13. kidney
14. pancreas
15. lower back
16. large intestine
17. appendix
18. small intestine
19. liver
20. stomach

21. chest
22. shoulder
23. oesophagus
24. mouth
25. spleen
26. neck
27. shoulder joint
28. trachea
29. heart
30. lung
31. brain point
32. clavicle
33. nose
34. testis (ovary)
35. forehead
36. tongue
37. eye
38. internal ear
39. tonsil

Acupoints of the ear showing corresponding internal organs

skin's surface, light movements have a major impact on the flow of lymph. Lymphatic drainage is always done towards the lymph nodes. In this sequence two or three fingers of each hand are used to gently sweep towards the lymph nodes located in the front of the ears, followed by sweeps down the sides of the face and neck, ending above the clavicles. These movements will channel lymph from the head and neck regions towards the two lymphatic ducts, where the fluid will be returned back to the bloodstream.

Ear massage

In 1957, Dr Paul Nogier, a physician from Lyon, France, developed a map of the outer ear based on the concept of an inverted foetus, with the head corresponding to the earlobe. Stimulation of the outer ear at locations corresponding to body parts is thought to have a beneficial effect on those organs. Each body organ or area has been mapped so a wide variety of problems can be treated. For this reason it is worthwhile taking time to massage the outer ears thoroughly. For your information we have included a diagram of the major points (above).

Start at the ear lobes, work your way up and down the ears using the thumb and index or middle finger. Travel up and down the ears three times for each of the movements.

Grounding

Having spent the complete treatment working on the head, it is important to bring the client's energy and awareness down to the lower parts of their body, otherwise they may feel lightheaded and a little 'spaced out'.

Sweeping down the arms and legs and gently holding the feet helps to ground the client.

After-treatment advice

See Chapter 6.

Massage sequence

Here is a suggested sequence for the massage following an ear candling treatment, but this can be adapted as you wish. Before beginning the massage, ensure that the client is comfortable. They may require a pillow or bolster under their knees to support the lower back. The use of oil is not necessary in this sequence, but you can use it if you choose to do so and if the client prefers this.

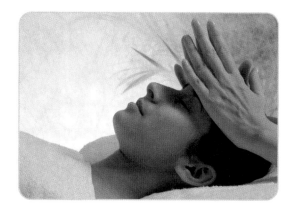

2 Effleurage face and neck starting from forehead

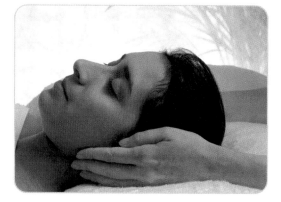

1 Gently place hands over the client's ears and hold for a few seconds. Slide hands to the top of the head and hold for a few seconds

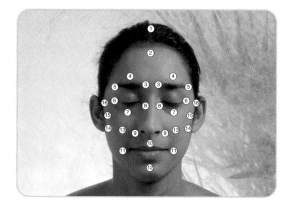

3 Pressure points: gently press all points indicated, 5 seconds on each point

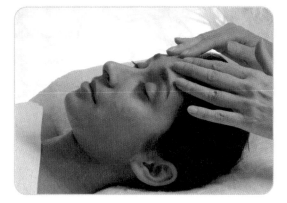

4 Friction: forehead, temples, cheeks using three fingers of each hand

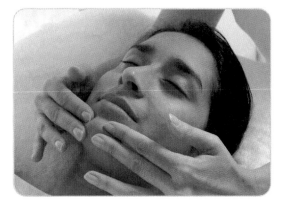

7 Friction: chin using three fingers of one hand, or two fingers of each hand

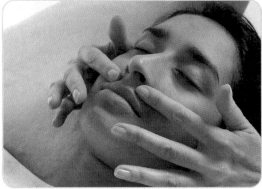

5 Friction: above mouth, using one finger of each hand

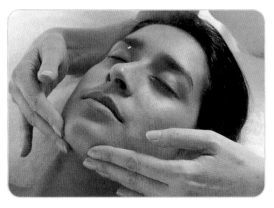

8 Friction: under jawbone using three fingers of each hand

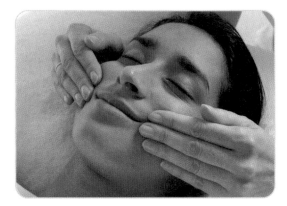

6 Friction: from sides of mouth outwards, then along jawbone using three fingers of each hand

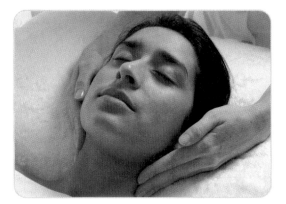

9 Friction: sides of neck using three fingers of each hand

79

ear candling in essence

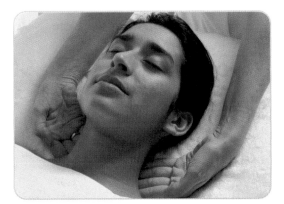

10 Friction: slide hands under back of neck and friction either side of spine

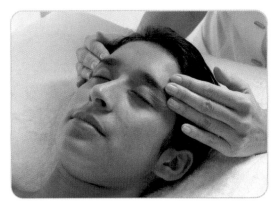

11 Lymphatic drainage from centre of forehead then down sides of neck three times

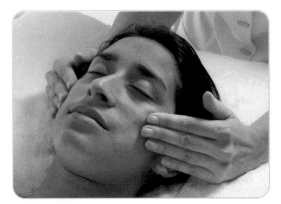

12 Lymphatic drainage along cheekbones then down sides of neck three times

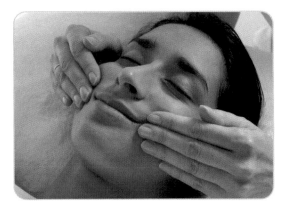

13 Lymphatic drainage down from sides of mouth then down sides of neck three times

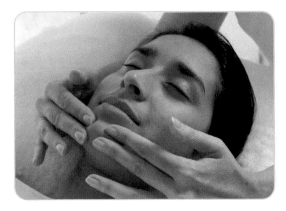

14 Lymphatic drainage along jaw bones then down sides of neck three times

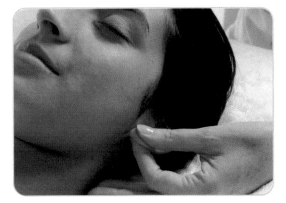

15 Squeeze ears starting at the lobes. Work up and down the ears three times

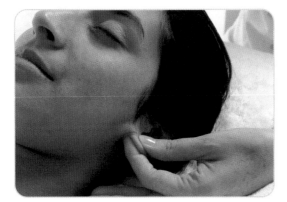

16 Friction: ears, starting at the lobes upwards. Work up and down three times

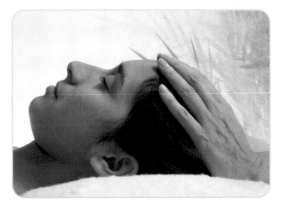

18 Head holding: Hold hands over the client's ears and hold for a few seconds. Hold hands on the crown and hold for a few seconds

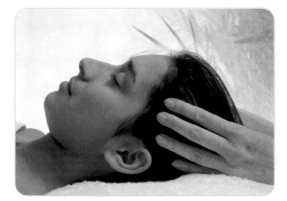

17 Friction: scalp, first behind ear lobes, then over top of scalp

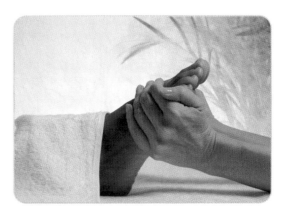

19 Grounding: sweep hands down sides of client's arms and legs three times. Hold client's feet for a few seconds

Following the treatment:

- Allow client to relax for a few minutes.
- Ask client to bend legs and sit up, and place their legs over side of couch.
- Squeeze shoulders and gently rub their back.

- Give client a glass of water.
- Assess effects of treatment and whether further treatments are required.
- Give client post-treatment advice (see p. 65).

FAQs

Can massage spread cancer around the body?

There is a lot of misinformation about massage and cancer. Many training organisations feel unable to recommend massage for cancer patients except in terminal stages of the disease because of the potential risk of metastases. However there is no researched evidence to show that this actually happens, and a lot of evidence to show the beneficial effects of massage. Our advice is that therapists wishing to work with cancer patients should take some extra training in this area and should never treat without consent from the clients' medical practitioner. Details of organisations that provide training courses for therapists wishing to work with cancer patients can be found in the useful addresses section.

What if my client does not like to have their face massaged?

It is important that the client rests for a while following the ear candling treatment and some form of massage can enhance the relaxation effects. Alternatives to the face massage include a hand or foot massage or a short reflexology treatment. If these are not appropriate, the client can simply relax on the treatment couch and listen to some gentle music. For safety reasons, it is best not to leave them unattended.

How much should the treatment cost?

The cost of the treatment will vary according to the location. The average cost for a 45 minute session including massage is £35.

anatomy and physiology

Anatomy is the science of the structure and make-up of the body, while physiology is the study of how the body functions. A sound knowledge of anatomy and physiology is very important for bodywork practitioners, who should have a complete knowledge of the structure and functions of each area on which they are working. In this chapter we examine the anatomy and physiology of the ear and associated structures, starting with the bones of the head.

The head

The head or skull is the most complex part of the human skeleton. It consists of two parts, the cranium and the face. It is composed of 22 bones, 21 of which are fused together at immovable joints called 'sutures' (the Latin word for stitches). The only moveable joint is the hinge-like temporomandibular joint (TMJ) in the jaw, connecting the bone in which our ears are located (temporal bone) with the lower jawbone (mandible).

The skull bones are classified into two groups. The eight cranial bones form the upper dome-shaped cranium which protects the brain and the organs of hearing, while the 14 facial bones provide attachment sites for the muscles of facial expression. The eye sockets or orbits and the nasal cavity are formed from both cranial and facial bones.

The cranial bones

- One frontal bone which forms the forehead, eye sockets and part of the nose.
- One occipital bone which forms the back of the skull and has a large opening called the 'foramen magnum' through which the spinal cord passes into the skull to join the brain.
- Two parietal bones which form the sides and roof of the cranium.

83

- Two temporal bones on each side of the head. These are the hardest bones in the body, with openings to the middle and inner ears.

- One butterfly-shaped sphenoid bone forming the floor of the cranium and with wings on either side forming the temples. The pituitary gland, which controls major bodily functions, is located in a small depression in the middle of the sphenoid bone.

- One rather complicated ethmoid bone containing several sections, most of which form the supporting structures of the nasal cavities. One of these sections is the 'cribriform plate', containing tiny holes through which nerves from the olfactory receptors (for sense of smell) in the nose pass to the brain. The ethmoid is a light spongy bone with several air-filled sinus cavities; hence its name which is derived from the Greek word 'ethmos' meaning 'sieve'.

The facial bones

- One mandible, commonly known as the lower jaw. This is the largest and strongest facial bone, and the only one that moves at the hinge-like temporomandibular joint (TMJ). One of the functions of this joint is to help expel earwax and prevent it from becoming compacted in the outer ear canal.

- Two maxillae, which form the upper jaw and the front part of the hard palate (roof of the mouth), part of the side walls of the nose and the floor of the orbits (eye sockets).

- Two palatine bones, which form the back part of the hard palate, part of the side walls of the nose and part of the floor of the orbits (eye sockets).

- Two small nasal bones, which form the bridge of the nose – the rest of the nose is composed of cartilage.

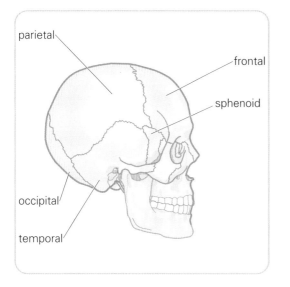

Bones of the cranium

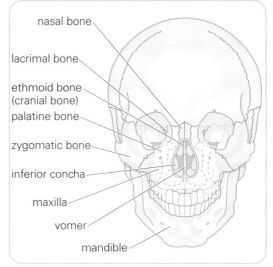

Bones of the face

- Two zygomatic bones which form the cheeks and the sides of the orbits
- Two tiny lacrimal bones, the size and shape of a little fingernail, on the inside walls of the orbits. A groove between the lacrimal bones and the nose forms a canal through which tears flow across the eyeball into the nasal cavity, leading to a 'runny nose' when crying.

- Two inferior conchae, which are scroll-like bones that form a curved ledge along the inside walls of the nasal cavity. They encourage the turbulent circulation and filtration of air before it passes into the lungs. Thus they are sometimes called 'turbinate bones'.
- One vomer which joins the ethmoid bone to form the nasal septum, which separates the two nostrils.

The ears and hearing – the auditory system

The ears are located in the temporal bones, and are the organs of both hearing and balance. We depend on our ears to help us interpret, communicate with and express the world around us. The human ear is fully developed at birth and responds to sounds that are very faint, as well as sounds that are very loud. Even in the womb, babies can respond to sound. Sounds can evoke sweet memories, calm and soothe a troubled mind, or trigger the release of powerful hormones preparing the body for fight or flight. Blind people make sense of their surroundings by tapping with a cane and listening carefully for the echoes. Sound begins with a movement, be it a voice, an engine or a bird shaking its feathers. This causes the air molecules all around it to tremble, then the molecules next to them tremble too, and the waves of sound continue to our ears where they are funnelled into the ear canal. The sound waves strike and rattle the eardrum, causing three tiny bones in the middle ear to move. This in turn presses fluid in the inner ear against membranes which brush tiny hairs; these trigger nerve cells nearby, carrying messages to the brain about what has been heard. This process is called the air conduction of sound. Sound travels through the air at 1,100 feet per second, much slower than the speed of light, which travels at 186,000 miles per second. That is why during a thunderstorm, the lightning can be seen before we hear the thunder roar.

Some sounds like our own voice or chewing crunchy food reaches the inner ear partly through the skull bones, a process called bone conduction. Sound waves travel faster through water than air, and fish and sea mammals are specially adapted to detect them. Whales emit a variety of sounds for communication and navigation underwater.

The ear has three distinct sections: the outer ear, the middle ear and the inner ear.

The outer ear

The outer ear consists of the pinna, a curvy flap of tissue on the side of the head, and the external auditory meatus or ear canal, which is about 2.5 cm long. The pinna is like a sound-gathering trumpet, funnelling sounds through the ear canal to reach the eardrum.

It is made of cartilage and soft tissue, so that it maintains its shape but is also pliable. Each little curve and hollow has its own name.

85

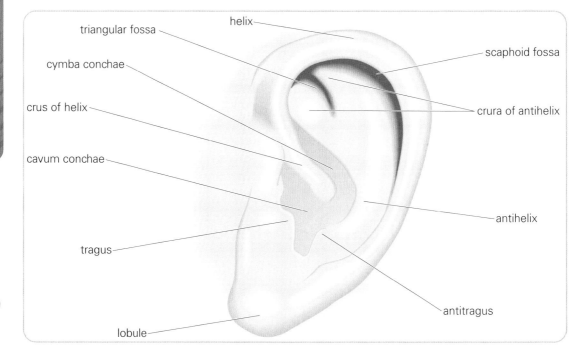

triangular fossa

helix

scaphoid fossa

cymba conchae

crus of helix

crura of antihelix

cavum conchae

antihelix

tragus

antitragus

lobule

Pinna of the ear

The part of the canal near the outside is cartilage covered with skin, while near the eardrum the wall of the canal becomes bony and is covered tightly by skin. The outer part of the ear canal has a profusion of hairs and around 4,000 glands that produce cerumen or earwax. These hairs trap dust and other potential irritants, while the wax protects the soft vulnerable skin that lines the ear canal and contains fatty acids that slow the growth of certain bacteria. It lubricates the eardrum and keeps it supple, and its bitter taste and smell also help keep insects out.

The eardrum (tympanic membrane) is a tightly stretched membrane, less than half an inch across. It is composed of three layers of tissue: an outer layer of hairless skin, a middle layer of fibrous tissue and an inner mucous membrane. When sound reaches the eardrum from the outside, it vibrates like a stick beating a drum. Even faint vibrations from a whisper can push it inwards ever so slightly. In an ear candling treatment, the sounds of the ingredients vapourising combined with the pressure waves from the vapours spiralling downwards, cause the eardrum to vibrate.

The middle ear

The middle ear is a space or cavity about 1.3cm across, filled with air. This cavity is connected with the nose and throat (naso-pharynx) by the Eustachian tube – also called the auditory tube (tuba auditiva). Named after an Italian anatomist, Bartolomeo Eustachio (1520–74), this tube is approximately 1.5 inches (36mm) long with a diameter of one-eighth to one quarter of an inch (3–6 mm). It is normally closed, but opens for 0.1 to 0.2 seconds during swallowing to allow air to move between the nasopharynx and middle ear (this equalises the pressure across the tympanic membrane). Changes in pressure outside the body, such as when flying in a plane or diving, cause the eardrum to bulge towards the area of lower pressure, and this can be painful. Swallowing, yawning or sucking help to equalise the pressure between the middle ear and the outside of the body by opening the Eustachian tube and allowing air into the middle ear. You can usually hear a popping sound as the Eustachian tube opens and the eardrum returns to its original position. In children, the Eustachian tube is shorter and straighter due to the facial and skull structure, so infections travel faster between middle ear, nose and throat.

The middle ear is also connected to air cells in the mastoid process, a projection of the temporal bone, which can be felt behind the ear. This channel is called the antrum and in some severe cases of middle ear infection, a mastoidectomy (removal of the mastoid process) may be necessary if the infection reaches this area. Fortunately mastoiditis (inflammation of the mastoid process) is uncommon these days, due to current day treatments.

Hinged together in the middle ear are three tiny bones, which conduct sound from the eardrum to the inner ear. These bones, the ossicles, are called the malleus, the incus and the stapes. You may also have heard them called the hammer, anvil and stirrup because they vaguely resemble those things.

The malleus is attached to the inner side of the eardrum, the incus stretches between the malleus and the stapes, and the base of the stapes fits against the oval window (a membrane separating the middle and the inner ear). When sound enters the ears and makes the eardrum vibrate, the vibrations pass from the eardrum along the ossicles. The stapes pushes like a little piston against the oval window, carrying the sound waves onwards.

The inner ear

The inner ear is a cavern hollowed out of the mastoid section of the temporal bone, and contains a maze of fluid-filled tubes. These bony tubes, the bony labyrinth, are filled with a fluid called perilymph. Within this bony labyrinth is a second series of delicate cellular tubes (a tube within a tube!) called the membranous labyrinth; this is filled with a fluid called endolymph. The inner ear has two membrane-covered outlets into the air-filled middle ear – the oval window and the round window. The oval window sits immediately behind the stapes, the third middle ear bone, and begins vibrating when struck by the stapes. This sets the fluid of the inner ear sloshing back and forth. The round window serves as a pressure valve, bulging outward as fluid pressure rises in the inner ear.

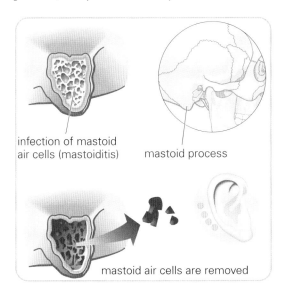

infection of mastoid air cells (mastoiditis)

mastoid process

mastoid air cells are removed

Infection of mastoid air cells – mastoiditis

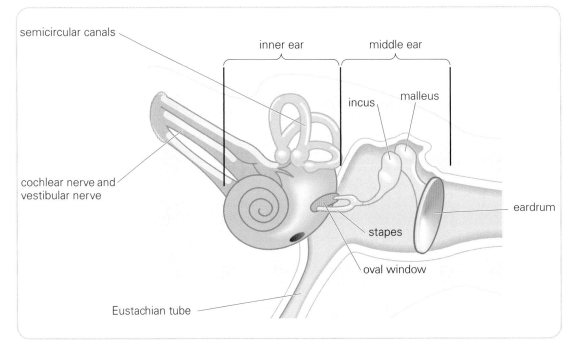

Structures of the middle and inner ear

The hearing component of the bony labyrinth is the snail-shaped cochlea, a spiral tube about 3.5cm long, which coils 2.7 times. This spiral tube contains two fluid-filled chambers, one within the other. The outer chamber starts at the oval window, continues to the tip of the cochlea and then doubles back, ending at the round window.

Sound vibrations cause the base of the stapes to rock to and fro against the oval window, agitating the perilymph in the outer chamber. At this point, the sound vibrations become fluid-borne rather than air borne. The vibrations are then transmitted to the endolymph in the inner chamber of the cochlea which contains a small structure called the Organ of Corti where the actual nerve cells for hearing are located. This sensitive element in the inner ear contains approximately 30,000 nerve cells and can be thought of as the body's microphone. These

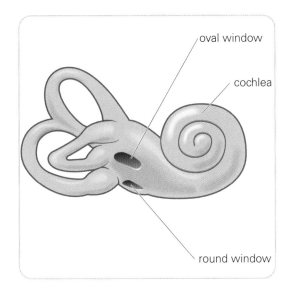

The cochlea

nerve cells are called hair cells because they have tiny hair-like structures called cilia, which project into the cochlear fluid. The hair

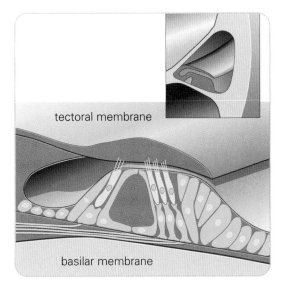

tectoral membrane

basilar membrane

Organ of Corti – the body's microphone

cells are connected to the cochlear nerve, a branch of the vestibulocochlear or auditory nerve (8th cranial nerve) which leads from the cochlea to the brain. This is actually two nerves joined together, the cochlear nerve for hearing and the vestibular nerve for equilibrium or balance.

When sound waves enter the cochlea, the cilia are moved, causing the hair cells to trigger an electrical impulse in the cochlear nerve. Different frequencies of sound are picked up by different hair cells, depending on where in the spiral tube they are located. The cochlear nerve passes electrical impulses to the brain, which recognizes them as sounds – such as people talking, or birds singing. Impulses arrive at a relay station in the mid–brain called the cochlear nucleus and from here, nerve fibres from each ear divide into two pathways. One pathway ascends straight to the auditory cortex on one side (hemisphere) of the brain. The other pathway crosses over and ascends to the auditory cortex on the other side (hemisphere) of the brain. As a result, each hemisphere of the brain receives information from both ears.

The ears and balance – the vestibular system

The balance component of the bony labyrinth is the vestibular system, which consists of three semi-circular canals, and two tiny sac-like structures called the utricle and the saccule.

While the semi-circular canals provide information about movement of the head, the sensory hair cells of the utricle and saccule provide information to the brain about head position when it is not moving. The functioning of the vestibular system depends on information from many systems including hearing, vision and information from the muscles.

The three semi-circular canals deal with dynamic equilibrium, which is the maintenance of the body's position (mainly the head) in response to sudden movements. They lie at right angles to one another and each deals with different movements: up and down, forward and backward, and tilting from one side to the other. All contain sensory hair cells that are activated by movement of inner ear fluid. As the body and head moves, hair cells in the semi-circular canals send nerve impulses to the brain by way of the vestibular portion of the auditory nerve (eighth cranial nerve). These nerve impulses are processed in the brain stem and cerebellum. This gives the brain information about the position of your head, helping to maintain your balance. For example, a sudden

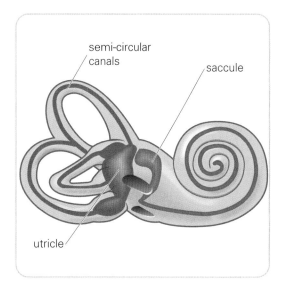

The semi-circular canals

loss of balance creates fluid movement in the semi-circular canals that triggers leg or arm reflex movements to restore balance.

Interconnecting the cochlea and the semi-circular canals is an area called the vestibule,

containing the utricle and the saccule, which are responsible for static equilibrium. They provide sensory information regarding the alignment of the head in relation to the ground (gravity) and are essential for maintaining posture as we sit or stand. They share the same fluid as the cochlea and semi-circular canals and have specialised hair cells called stereocilia, connected to the brain by the vestibular portion of the auditory nerve. When you move your head, the stereocilia are moved, triggering an electrical impulse in the vestibular nerve; this relays the information to the cerebellum of the brain.

The cerebellum sends messages to the motor area of the cerebrum in the brain, which in turn sends messages to the skeletal muscles, controlling posture.

Since the ears, nose and throat are all intimately connected, it is very easy for infection to travel from one to the other; so we will briefly look at these other structures.

The nose

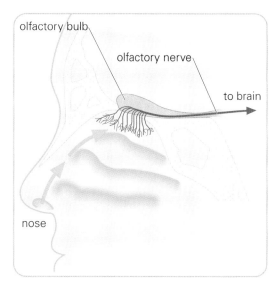

The nose is the entry point for air into the body, warming and moistening the air as it passes through. It has tiny hairs called cilia that filter dust particles, while its mucous lining traps bacteria and particles that get past the hairs. A new mucous lining is produced every 20 minutes, while the cilia whip the old mucous back to the throat to be swallowed. Stomach acid kills the bacteria so that it does not cause us any harm.

The other major job of the nose is the detection of odours, which is accomplished by nerve endings in the roof of the nose. Odour molecules float back into the nasal cavity where they are picked up by some of the ten million receptor cells, which fire impulses to the brain's smell centre. The nerve endings in the nose are unique in that they are replaced about every 30 days, unlike other nerves in the body which are not replaced when damaged.

The sinuses

Opening into the nasal passages are the paranasal sinuses, cavities or air pockets located inside the bones in the skull.

- ⚬ The two maxillary sinuses are around the area of the cheeks. These two sinuses are present at birth and continue to grow as the bones develop.

- ⚬ The ethmoid sinuses are located around the area of the bridge of the nose, behind and in between the eyes. They are also present at birth.

- ⚬ In the forehead are the frontal sinuses, which do not develop until around seven years of age.

- ⚬ The sphenoid sinuses are located deep in the face, behind the nose, and do not develop until adolescence.

As well as giving resonance to the voice, the sinuses warm and moisten the air as we inhale, and help to reduce the weight of the skull. Like the nose, they are lined with very fine hair-like cilia whose function is to move the mucus normally produced by the sinuses towards a tiny hole (ostium) about the size of a pin hole, which provides drainage for the sinus into the nasal cavity.

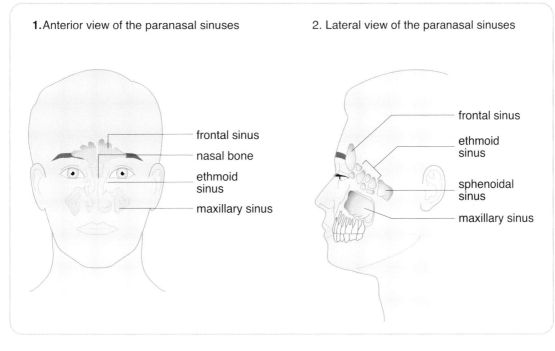

1. Anterior view of the paranasal sinuses

frontal sinus
nasal bone
ethmoid sinus
maxillary sinus

2. Lateral view of the paranasal sinuses

frontal sinus
ethmoid sinus
sphenoidal sinus
maxillary sinus

Anterior and lateral view of paranasal sinuses

Sinusitis

Sinusitis occurs when the paranasal sinuses become inflamed, either acutely or as a chronic condition. Acute sinusitis can occur as the result of an infection by bacteria or virus, or as the result of inflammation caused by allergy; it may last from one day to three weeks.

Inflammation of the nasal passages due to an upper respiratory tract infection may also produce sinusitis, as secretions are unable to drain freely. When sinusitis occurs frequently, i.e. more than four times per year, or persists for three months, it is described as chronic sinusitis and in this instance is more likely to be due to allergy or mixed bacterial infection.

casestudy

Practitioner Lesley's story demonstrates the positive effects of ear candling in alleviating sinus problems:

'Maureen, aged 73, suffered with chronic sinus problems on a daily basis – tenderness in the cheeks, pain around the eyes, headaches, and congestion, particularly on the left side. Initially, she had three treatments on a weekly basis. During the first treatment she felt a popping sensation in the head, and felt the flow of mucous. The treatment gave immediate relief, ie her airways felt clearer and she described her head as feeling "lighter". There was lots of wax and residue in the candles, particularly on the left side. Further improvement was experienced after the second treatment, and by the third treatment the symptoms had improved dramatically. She had not experienced headaches or pain around her eyes since treatment one, her airways felt clearer, the tenderness in her cheeks significantly reduced, and she felt more energised. Maureen said that the treatments "have changed my life".'

The throat

The throat is a ring-like muscular tube that acts as the passageway for air, food and liquid, as well as helping to form speech. The throat, which is divided into three sections, is also called the pharynx. It consists of:

- the naso-pharynx behind the nose
- the oro-pharynx at the back of the mouth, behind the tonsils
- the laryngo-pharynx or larynx (also known as the voice box), composed of cartilage, muscles, and soft tissue which contains the vocal cords.

The vocal cords are the upper opening into the windpipe (trachea), the passageway to the lungs.

A flap of soft tissue called the epiglottis is located just above the vocal cords. It folds down over the trachea to prevent food and irritants from entering the lungs when eating.

The tonsils and adenoids, composed of lymphatic tissue, are located at the back and the sides of the mouth to protect against infection entering the body via the mouth. Upper respiratory infections can cause them to become inflamed and swollen.

A small isolated U-shaped bone called the hyoid is located in the neck, below and supporting the tongue. It is held in position by muscles and ligaments, which attach it to the temporal bone. If you put your hand to the front of your throat and swallow, you can feel the hyoid bone move up and down.

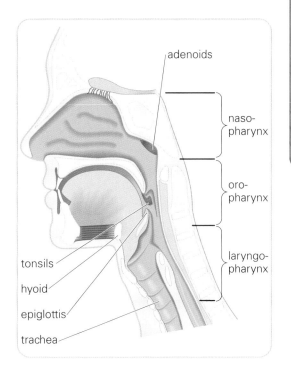

Internal structure of the throat

Hearing problems

Deafness can have many complex causes but is divided into two main types:

- conductive deafness – where sound cannot be conducted freely through the outer or middle ear
- sensorineural deafness – where the cause of the deafness is in the cochlea or in the hearing nerve.

A build-up of compacted earwax in the outer ear canal is the most common cause of conductive deafness. It can also be caused by a foreign body in the ear canal, and as we become older the eardrum gradually thickens, leading to age-related deafness. Other causes of conductive deafness include the following:

Otosclerosis

This is caused by a bony overgrowth of the stapes, one of the bones in the chain which stretches across the middle ear. The link in the chain becomes rigid and sound vibrations cannot pass through it. People with otosclerosis gradually become more deaf. This condition affects more women than men. It can run in families and often begins around the age of 30. Sufferers often use hearing aids until it becomes very severe, and then the option is a stapedectomy, where a tiny peg replaces the stapes so that sound can travel to the inner ear. This operation has a high success rate.

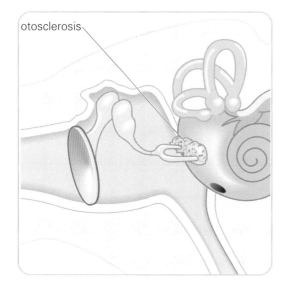

otosclerosis

Otosclerosis

Damaged ossicles

Serious infections and head injuries can damage or displace the bones of the middle ear, and occasionally babies are born with malformed ossicles. They can be repaired or replaced by having an operation called an ossiculoplasty. Cranial osteopathy can sometimes realign misplaced ossicles and improve hearing.

Perforated eardrums

This can be caused by untreated otitis media (middle ear infection) or other serious infections, head injuries, explosions or poking things in the ear. The larger the perforation, the greater the loss of hearing. The location of the hole (perforation) in the eardrum also affects the degree of hearing loss. If the perforated eardrum is due to a sudden traumatic or explosive event, the loss of hearing can be great and ringing in the ear (tinnitus) may be severe. In this case the hearing usually returns partially and the ringing diminishes in a few days. Chronic infection as a result of the perforation can cause major hearing loss. Perforated eardrums normally heal by themselves and any hearing loss is usually temporary. More serious damage can be treated by an operation called a myringoplasty (tympanoplasty), in which a tissue graft is used to seal up the hole.

Cholesteatoma

This is a skin growth that occurs in the middle ear behind the eardrum. It is usually due to repeated infection, which causes an ingrowth of the skin of the eardrum. Cholesteatomas often take the form of a cyst or pouch that sheds layers of old skin building up inside the ear. Over time, the cholesteatoma can increase in size and destroy the surrounding delicate bones of the middle ear. Hearing loss, dizziness and facial muscle paralysis can result from continued cholesteatoma growth. The condition usually occurs because of poor Eustachian tube function, as well as infection in the middle ear. When the Eustachian tubes are malfunctioning due to allergy, a cold or sinusitis, the air in the middle ear is absorbed by the body, leading to a partial vacuum. The vacuum pressure sucks in a pouch or sac by stretching the eardrum, especially areas weakened by previous infections. This sac often becomes a cholesteatoma.

Initially, the ear may drain, sometimes with a bad odour. As the cholesteatoma pouch enlarges, it can cause a full feeling in the ear, along with hearing loss. Dizziness or muscle weakness of the face on the side of the infected ear can also occur. Anyone suffering from any or all of these symptoms should seek a medical investigation. Treatment may consist of a careful cleaning of the ear, medication, and eardrops to control the infection, but large cholesteatomas usually require surgical removal.

Sensorineural deafness

This is most often the result of damage to tiny hair cells in the cochlea. These hair cells cannot be replaced, and hearing loss is permanent.

People with sensorineural deafness usually find hearing aids very helpful. A cochlear implant may be an option for people who have become profoundly deaf through sensorineural deafness, or for children who are born deaf. Better results are likely if this is done while they are still very young. A cochlear implant is a small electronic device, part of which is implanted in the cochlea and part of which is worn externally (see diagram on p 52). It does not give perfect hearing, but many people who have cochlear implants can understand speech and recognise different sounds around them. Some people with cochlear implants can also use the telephone.

There are many causes of sensorineural deafness including the following, all of which can damage the cochlear hair cells:

- A disease such as mumps or meningitis.

- Certain strong drugs, in particular platinum-based chemotherapy drugs, or antibiotics called aminoglycosides – eg streptomycin and gentamicin.

- Long-term exposure to loud noise. By law, if you work somewhere very noisy you must be given earplugs or muffs to protect your hearing. Cochlear hair cells can be irrevocably damaged by just a single exposure to a very loud noise.

- A serious head injury with a skull fracture.

- The ageing process – presbyacusis is the name given to the hearing loss many people experience in old age. Everyone loses hair cells in the cochlea throughout their life, and gradually hearing becomes less sharp. Those with presbyacusis may find that people seem to mumble, and they often find it difficult to understand what is being said, especially in noisy places. Properly fitted hearing aids are usually helpful.

- Before a baby is born, if the mother has rubella (German measles) while pregnant, or to a baby following a premature birth or difficult labour.

- Sensorineural deafness from birth may also be genetic and it is common for members of the same family to have the same pattern of hearing loss as they get older.

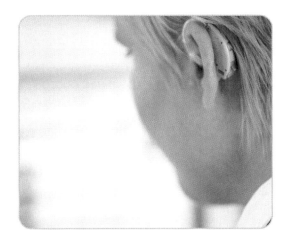

A typical hearing aid

Balance problems

There are many medical conditions that may make you feel dizzy. Few of them are serious, but it is a good idea to have the specific cause of your dizziness diagnosed and treated. Balance problems and dizziness can be treated in several ways, such as taking a course of prescribed drugs, or using a set of balance-retraining exercises. Even when a balance problem is taking a long time to improve, there is almost always a course of treatment that will help.

Causes of dizziness and balance problems include the following:

Blood pressure

Low blood pressure can cause a light-headed sensation. On standing up, blood tends to pool in the veins of the legs. This is stopped by nerves which contract the veins in the legs, ensuring that enough blood returns to the heart and that there is no reduction in the amount of blood that the heart pumps to the brain. However, if there is pooling of blood in the veins, less blood returns to the heart and less is pumped out, which means a reduction in the amount of blood going to the brain. This causes symptoms of dizziness and some people may faint. This occasionally happens, for example, to palace guards when they have been standing in one position for too long. If you have low blood pressure and you also have symptoms of dizziness or faintness when standing up suddenly, you should have your blood pressure checked, both when you are lying down and when you then stand up. This drop in blood pressure when you stand up is called postural hypotension. Many people naturally have quite low blood pressure, which causes no problems. In fact, they are protected from the effects of salt and other factors that can cause raised blood pressure levels and on average, they are healthier and live longer than those with higher blood pressure.

Menière's disease

This is caused by increased pressure of the fluid in the inner ear. The symptoms include sensorineural deafness, tinnitus and vertigo. During bouts of Menière's disease, the dizziness may make it difficult to walk or stand, and there may be vomiting. Bouts happen at intervals – there may be weeks or years between them. Deafness and tinnitus may become better and worse at different times. Sufferers are usually advised to follow a special low-salt diet, as excess salt encourages fluid retention in the body. Certain medication such as a diuretic (water pill) or anti-vertigo medication can also help. Stress may aggravate the vertigo and tinnitus of Menière's disease.

Tinnitus

This is a condition whereby noises such as buzzing, ringing, whistling, hissing and other sounds are heard in the ears or in the head. There are many different causes of tinnitus. It can be linked to exposure to loud noise, hearing loss, injuries to the ear or head, compacted earwax, some diseases of the ear or emotional stress. It can also be a side effect of medication, or a combination of all of the above. Many people with tinnitus have never had any of these and do not have a hearing loss.

casestudy

The following case study was sent to us by practitioner Linda:

'Tricia, aged 62, had been suffering from severe tinnitus for about a month. The tinnitus was worse in the left ear. She has diverticulitis, which is controlled by regular reflexology. She had three treatments of ear candling on a fortnightly basis. After the first treatment there was wax and powder residue in both candles. The right candle took nine minutes to burn and the left candle took 10 minutes. After the first treatment the tinnitus symptoms were significantly reduced, particularly in the right ear. On the second treatment the candles took nine minutes to burn down on both sides. During the treatment Tricia experienced a popping sensation in both ears. At the end of the treatment there was no ringing noise in either ear. There was still wax and powder residue in both candles. After about an hour a slight noise came back in the left side. The next day the noise in the ears returned and got much worse for four days; this was a "healing crisis", ie the symptoms became worse before improving. After four days, the tinnitus then eased off considerably. After treatment three, there was no noise in the right and only a slight noise in the left ear. The severe symptoms she was experiencing before her first candling treatment have not returned, and she was so impressed with the way that ear candling can reduce tinnitus symptoms that she trained as an ear candling therapist.'

FAQs

What is motion sickness?

Dizziness, vertigo and motion sickness all relate to the sense of balance. The sense of balance is maintained by a complex interaction of:

- the inner ears, which monitor the directions of motion
- the eyes, which monitor where the body is in space (ie upside down etc) as well as directions of motion
- skin pressure receptors such as those in the joints and spine, which tell what part of the body is down and touching the ground
- the muscle and joint sensory receptors, which tell what parts of the body are moving

- the central nervous system which processes all the bits of information from the four other systems to make sense out of it all.

The symptoms of motion sickness and dizziness appear when the central nervous system receives conflicting messages from the other four systems. For example, suppose you are sitting in the back seat of a moving car reading a book. Your inner ears and skin receptors will detect the motion of your travel, but your eyes see only the pages of your book. You could become 'car sick'.

What can I do for motion sickness?

- Always ride where your eyes will see the same motion that your body and inner ears feel. For example, sit in the front seat of the car and look at the distant scenery; go up on the deck of the ship and watch the horizon; sit by the window in an aeroplane and look outside.

- Do not read while travelling and do not sit in a seat facing backward if you suffer from motion sickness.
- Do not watch or talk to another traveller who is having motion sickness.
- Avoid strong odours and spicy or greasy foods immediately before and during your travel.

What can I do to reduce dizziness?

- Avoid rapid changes in position, especially from lying down to standing up or turning around from one side to the other.
- Avoid extremes of head motion (especially looking up) or rapid head motion (especially turning or twisting).
- Eliminate or decrease the use of products that impair circulation, eg nicotine, caffeine and salt.
- Minimise your exposure to circumstances that precipitate your dizziness, such as stress and anxiety or substances to which you are allergic.
- Avoid hazardous activities when you are dizzy, such as driving or operating dangerous equipment.

Are there any natural remedies to help with dizziness or balance problems?

If your fluid balance is not good, drink more water and avoid nicotine, caffeine and fizzy drinks as these decrease blood flow to the brain. Cut down on salt as this encourages water retention and leads to poor circulation.

If the inner ear fails to receive enough blood flow, a more specific type of dizziness called vertigo (a spinning sensation) occurs. The inner ear is very sensitive to minor alterations of blood flow and all of the causes for poor circulation to the brain also apply specifically to the inner ear. The herb ginkgo biloba improves blood supply to the head so will help ear conditions caused by poor circulation. This herb also improves memory, but those who are on anti-coagulant drugs should not take it.

Other recommended herbal remedies include vinca minor, which has similar effects to ginkgo biloba without the contraindications with anticoagulants. Valerian may help to reduce stress and tension that are causing constriction in the head and neck. Taking a supplement of Co-enzyme Q10 is thought to help with Menière's disease. *Before taking any natural remedies for dizziness or balance problems, it is very important to check with your doctor and seek advice from a qualified herbalist, as some herbal remedies may react with your medication.*

where to go from here

Continuing professional development (CPD) is the means by which members of professional associations maintain, improve and broaden their knowledge and skills, and develop the personal qualities required in their professional lives. Continuing professional development is an essential part of lifelong learning and career development. Lifelong learning was identified by the government as essential for all people over the age of 16 years. This is reflected in Government White papers such as 'A First Class Service – Quality in the New NHS' (1998) where importance is attached to CPD for all National Health Service staff, whether qualified or unqualified.

CPD has always applied to doctors, lawyers, accountants, financial advisers etc, and nowadays it also applies to complementary therapists and beauty therapists who wish to keep their expertise up to date with current developments. Most professional organisations require their members to undertake a minimum number of CPD hours annually. Even without this requirement, it is very important to keep up to date on trends in the industry and to update your skills, whatever your line of work.

CPD maintains high professional standards through increased knowledge and awareness. It is also good marketing for your practice and will add to your client base!

Courses in ear candling are offered as CPD for therapists, and this is an ideal treatment to add to your repertoire. For the therapist the advantages of learning how to practise ear candling include:

- it does not take long to learn – most courses are for one day
- it is pleasant and relaxing to perform – you remain seated during the treatment
- client satisfaction is very rewarding.

Topics covered on an ear candling course will include:

- history and background of the treatment
- benefits

- contraindications
- types of ear candles used and how they work
- anatomy and physiology of the ear and related structures
- how to carry out the treatment (practical session)
- analysis of treatment.

FAQs: About ear candling courses

What are the prerequisites to receiving a professional qualification in ear candling?

Ear candling courses are usually postgraduate courses, suitable for qualified therapists (complementary and beauty therapists) and those working within the health services. On successful completion of the course, a certificate of competence will allow them to practise this holistic treatment on their clients and others. Check with the individual course provider regarding the prerequisites for their courses, as these may differ.

Will my insurance premium be higher if I wish to practise ear candling?

As a practising therapist you should have professional indemnity and public liability insurance, and most policies incorporate these two elements. The former protects you in the event of a claim of personal injury or damage resulting from a treatment you carried out. The latter covers you if a member of the public is injured on your premises or if their property is damaged. If

you are running a business where you employ people and you sell products, you will also need to have employer's liability and product liability insurance. Some insurers (but not all) charge an extra premium to cover ear candling, and regard it as a slightly higher risk due to the fact that an open flame is used. You will need to contact your insurer to check if they charge an extra premium. Just as you shop around for your home and car insurance, it is worth shopping around for insurance to cover you as a therapist, and we have included some addresses on the following pages.

I am not a qualified therapist but I would like to do an ear candling course so that I can practise it safely on my family. Is this possible?

You will need to check with the course provider about this. Ear candles are now readily available to members of the public and many people use them at home, so some course providers do accept non-therapists on courses.

Useful addresses

Ear candling training courses

Hands on Training:
Tel +44 (0) 18 9272 5716
Website: www.hands-on-training.net
Email: linda_ayers@hotmail.com

For courses held in the UK and internationally:
Lesley Hart
Tel +44 (0) 20 8462 1886 or +44 (0) 1892 725716
Email: lesleyphart@yahoo.co.uk
Website: www.hands-on-training.net

For courses held in the UK, Ireland and internationally
Mary Dalgleish
Tel +44 (0) 20 8874 9047
Email: marydalgleish@yahoo.co.uk
Website: www.head2toemassage.co.uk

Other ear candling courses

- www.itecworld.co.uk
- www.vtct.co.uk
- www.hotcourses.com
- www.healthypages.net

Find an ear candling therapist

- www.hands-on-training.net
- www.the-cma.org.uk
- www.embodyprofessional.com

- www.fht.org.uk
- www.iptiuk.com
- www.healthypages.net

Insurance for ear candling:

- www.towergategroup.co.uk
- www.iptiuk.com
- www.balen.co.uk
- www.babtac.com
- www.embodyprofessional.com
- www.fht.org.uk

Suppliers

International supplier of Hopi ear candles
BIOSUN GmbH
35641 Schwalbach
PO Box 100
Germany
Phone: +49 64 45 / 60 07 - 0
Email: info@biosun.com
Website: www.biosun.de

UK distributor of BIOSUN Hopi ear candles
Revital Ltd
Unit D3, Braintree Industrial Estate
Braintree Road
Ruislip
Middlesex HA4 0EJ
Tel: +44 (0) 8 8454118
Customer service: 0870 366 5729
Mail order hotline: 0800 252 875
Website: www.revital.com

OTOSAN ear cones
For UK distributors contact:
Malozza Distribution Ltd
PO Box 184
Whitstable, Kent CT5 3WF
Tel: 0870 4211718
Email: sales@malozzadistribution.com

For international distributors see
www.otosan.com

Ear candling treatment cloths
Hands on Training
Tel: 01892 725716
email: linda_ayers@hotmail.com
www.hands-on-training.net

Ear poppers
Micromedics (USA)
Tel: 001 800 624 5662
Website: www.earpopper.com

Related associations

Menière's Society
The Rookery
Surrey Hills Business Park
Dorking
Surrey RH5 6QT
Tel: 0845 120 2975
Website: www.menieres.org.uk

British Tinnitus Association
Ground Floor
Unit 5
Acorn Business Park
Woodseats Close
Sheffield S8 0TB
Tel: 0114 250 9922
Website: www.tinnitus.org.uk

The Cancer Resource Centre
20–22 York Road
London SW11 3QT
Tel: 020 7924 3924
Website: www.cancer-resource-centre.org.uk

British Society of Audiology
80 Brighton Road
Reading
Berks RG6 1PS
Tel: 01189 660622
Website: www.thebsa.org.uk

RNID (Royal National Institute of the Deaf)
19–23 Featherstone Street
London EC1Y 8SL
Telephone: 020 7296 8000
Textphone: 020 7296 8001
Website: www.rnid.org.uk

The Prince of Wales's Foundation for
Integrated Health
33–41 Dallington Street
London EC1V 0BB
Tel: 020 3119 3100
Fax: 020 3119 3101
Email: info@fih.org.uk
Website: www.fih.org.uk

Other Addresses

Dr Antony Mathews
Consultant Osteopathic Ototogist
Herne Bay Osteopathic Clinic
70 Canterbury Road
Herne Bay
Kent CT6 5SB
Tel: 01227-366473
Email: Antony-Mathews@
hernebayosteopathic.freeserve.co.uk

Kirlian photography
Anne-Marie Cogdell
Tel: 01689 854359
Email: sphereii@tiscali.co.uk

Bibliography and further reading

Brennan, Barbara Ann (1987) *Hands of Light*, Bantam Books, USA

Cohen, S (1987) *The Magic of Touch*, Harper & Row, New York, NY

Davis, P (1991) *Subtle Aromatherapy*, CW Daniel, UK

Field, T, PhD (2001) *Touch*, the MIT Press, Cumberland, RI

Hamilton, Jili (2004) *Hopi Candles*, Pen Press, London

Hix, Sue (1998) *Fourteen Classical Meridian Charts for Shiatsu, Energy Healing & Martial Arts*, Rosewell Publications, UK

Holford, P (2002) *The Optimum Nutrition Bible*, Piatkus Publishers Ltd, London

Looker, T and Gregson, O (2003) *Managing Stress*, Hodder Headline, UK

Maab, Dr C, Jung, Dr K, Funke-Leschik, C (1998) *Complex Therapy of Tinnitus*, BIOSUN publication, Germany

McNamara, P (1977) *Massage for People with Cancer*, Wandsworth Cancer Resource Centre, London

McGuinness Helen (2002) *Anatomy & Physiology Therapy Basics*, Hodder & Stoughton, UK

Moberg, K (2003) *The Oxytocin Factor*, De Capo Press, Cambridge, MA

Montagy, A (1986) *Touching*, Harper & Row, New York, NY

Ozaniec, Naomi (1991) *The Elements of the Chakras*, Element Books, UK

Pert, Canduce B, PhD (1997) *Molecules of Emotion*, Simon & Schuster, UK

Parliament publications: *Sixth report, 21 November 2000 by the Select Committee appointed to consider Science and Technology. Ordered to report: complementary and alternative medicine.* The Stationery Office, UK

Prince of Wales's Foundation for Integrated Health (2005) *Complementary Healthcare, a Guide for Patients*, UK

Reiner, Dr Heidi (2002) *Statistical assessment of an Application Observation with BIOSUN Ear candles in typical areas of application (secondary effects of colds, headaches, ear aches, ear noises and stress)*, BIOSUN publication, Germany

Riza Centre of National Medicine, Milan (1992) *Use of OTOSAN Ear cones in the presence of excess earwax and use of OTOSAN Ear Cones in cases of otalgia in children*

Ross and Wilson, Anne Waugh and Allison Grant (2001) *Anatomy and Physiology in Health and Illness*, Churchill Livingstone, Edinburgh

Rutherford, Leo (2001) *Your Shamanic Path*, Piatkus Publishers Ltd, London

Sceats, Andrew (2004) *Ear Candling & Other Treatments for Ear, Nose & Throat Problems*, Pressuredown Therapies, UK

Siegfried, Donna Rae (2002) *Anatomy & Physiology for Dummies*, Wiley Publishing Inc., New York

Tortora G and Grabowski R (1990) *Principles of Anatomy and Physiology*, Harper Row Publishers, New York

Wood, Nicholas (2001) *The Book of the Shaman*, Barron's, New York, NY

Oxford Minidictionary for Nurses (1998) Oxford University Press, UK

Websites

www.rnid.org.uk
www.patient.co.uk
www.fih.org.uk
http://en.wikipedia.org
www.biosun.de
www.otosan.com
http://www.parliament.the-stationery-office.

co.uk/pa/ld199900/ldselect/ldsctech/123/
12302.htm
www.Rosewellshiatsu.co.uk
www.cancer-resource-centre.org.uk
www.therapists-r-us.com
www.bristolcancerhelp.org
www.healer.ch

Glossary

Allergens: Substances that cause an allergic response in some individuals, and may affect the upper respiratory system causing a runny nose, watery, itchy eyes, or wheezing. Allergens are present in saliva, urine and small particles of feathers or hair from warm-blooded animals such as dogs, cats, birds, and rodents. They are also present in grass pollen, mould spores or house dust mite faeces (present in dust). Other allergens may affect the skin or the digestive system.

Aminoglycosides: A group of strong antibiotics (such as gentamicin) that are used against certain types of bacteria.

Analgesic: A compound that can alleviate pain.

Anthropologists: Anthropologists study people and primates (such as chimps), researching their cultural, physical, and social development over time.

Antioxidants: A substance that prevents damage to cells of the body caused by free radicals. Free radicals are highly reactive chemicals which can destroy cells, and they play a role in many diseases. Vitamins A, C, E and some of the B vitamins, beta-carotene, selenium and some key enzymes in your body are all antioxidants. By intercepting the free radicals, antioxidants prevent them from damaging molecular structures such as your DNA.

Apnoea: The temporary cessation of breathing from any cause.

Aristotle: Aristotle (384–322 BC) was an ancient Greek philosopher. He and Plato are considered to be the most influential philosophers in Western thought. He wrote many books about physics, poetry, zoology, government, and biology.

Auditory cortex: The area of the brain (in the temporal cortex) that connects with fibres from the auditory nerve and interprets nerve impulses in a form that is perceived as sound.

Aura: An emanation of energy, which surrounds all living things. People with psychic abilities are able to see and interpret this energy.

Autoimmune: A condition in which the immune system attacks the body's own tissues. To function properly, the immune system must identify foreign substances such as bacteria, viruses, parasites, etc, and it must be able to distinguish normal body tissue from these foreign substances. If it fails to distinguish the difference, it attempts to destroy the tissue it wrongly identifies as foreign. For example, in rheumatoid arthritis, the body attacks the synovial lining of its own joints.

Barotrauma: This is a condition of discomfort in the ear caused by pressure differences between the inside and the outside of the eardrum. The air pressure in the middle ear is usually the same as the air pressure outside of the body. If the Eustachian tube running between the middle ear and the back of the throat is blocked, the air pressure in the middle ear is different from the pressure on the outside of the eardrum, causing barotrauma. Barotrauma commonly occurs with altitude changes such as when flying, scuba diving, or driving in the mountains. If you have a congested nose from allergies, colds, or upper respiratory infection, barotrauma is more likely.

Blood pressure: This refers to the force of blood exerted on the inside walls of blood vessels. Blood pressure is expressed as a ratio (eg 120/80 is normal blood pressure for a healthy adult). The first number is the *systolic* pressure, or the pressure when the heart is pushing blood out into the arteries. The second number is the *diastolic* pressure, or the pressure when the heart is resting and filling with blood. High blood pressure is called *hypertension* and low blood pressure is called *hypotension*.

Cancer: Any malignant growth or tumour caused by abnormal and uncontrolled cell division; it may grow directly into other tissues (invasion) or spread to other parts of the body through the lymphatic system or the blood stream (metastasis).

Carcinogenic: Capable of causing cancer.

Cardiovascular system: The system composed of the heart, blood vessels, and blood.

Cartilage: A fibrous connective tissue that lines joints and helps form the flexible portions of the nose and the ears.

Carotenoids: Natural fat-soluble pigments found in certain plants. They provide the bright red, orange, or yellow colour of many vegetables, serve as antioxidants, and can be a source for vitamin A activity.

Cerebellum: A large portion of the base of the brain between the cerebrum and the brain stem. It is responsible for the coordination of voluntary movements, posture, and balance and is located in the back of the skull behind the brainstem.

Cerebral palsy: A general term for a group of permanent brain injuries as a result of an episode that causes a lack of oxygen to the brain while in the womb, during birth, or in the months following birth. It is a lifelong condition that affects the communication between the brain and the muscles, causing a permanent state of uncoordinated movement and posturing.

Cerebrum: The largest portion of the brain, divided into two hemispheres (halves) which each contains four lobes. Its functions include speech, memory, vision, personality and muscle control in certain parts of the body. One of the lobes on each side is the temporal lobe containing an area called the auditory cortex, which is necessary for interpreting sounds.

Cerumen: Commonly known as earwax, cerumen is a yellowish, waxy substance secreted by ceruminous glands in the ear canal of humans and many other mammals. It plays a vital role in the human ear canal, assisting in cleaning and lubrication, and also provides a degree of protection from bacteria, fungus, and insects that dislike its bitter taste and smell.

Chemotherapy: The treatment of cancer using specific drugs intended to destroy malignant cells and tissues. Chemotherapy may be taken by mouth or it may be put into the body by a needle inserted into a vein or muscle.

Chickenpox: An acute, contagious viral disease, usually contracted by young children. The infection is characterised by a fever and itchy, red spots usually appearing on the chest and stomach first, then appearing in crops over the entire body. The red spots turn into small blisters that dry up and form scabs over about a week. They occasionally cause scarring (particularly if scratched) or if they become infected with bacteria. Shingles or herpes zoster is the adult form of chickenpox, caused by the same virus (varcella-zoster) due to infection of the posterior roots of the spinal nerves or the fifth cranial nerve. It is marked by a painful eruption of blisters, usually on one side of the body along the course of one or more nerves.

Clairvoyant: A person with the ability to see subtle energy, ie the ability to see the aspects of the aura such as its size, shape, chakras and colours.

Cleopatra: (69–30 BC) Cleopatra was the beautiful and charismatic queen of Egypt; mistress of Julius Caesar and later of Mark Anthony. She killed herself to avoid capture by Octavian, Julius Caesar's grandnephew and adopted son.

Cochlear implant: An electronic medical device surgically implanted in the inner ear which bypasses the hair cells of the cochlea and directly stimulates the auditory nerve to send signals to the brain. The two external components of the device are a headpiece receiver/microphone and a speech processor.

Conjunctivitis: Commonly known as 'pink eye', this is an inflammation of the membrane (conjunctiva) that covers the eye and lines the inner surface of the eyelid. The main causes of conjunctivitis are bacterial or viral infections, irritants such as air pollutants, smoke, soap, hairspray, make-up, chlorine or cleaning fluids and seasonal allergic response to grass and other pollens. There is normally itching, redness, sensitivity to light, feeling as if something is in the eye, swelling of the lids and discharge from the eyes. It usually takes from a few days to two weeks for most types of conjunctivitis to clear. Medications in the form of ointments, drops or pills may be recommended to help kill the germ infecting the eye, relieve allergic symptoms and decrease discomfort. In the case of conjunctivitis due to a viral cold or flu, the practitioner may recommend that you be patient and let it run its course.

Cranio-sacral osteopathy: Cranio-sacral is the name given to the approach to osteopathy developed by Dr WG Sutherland, a hundred years ago in America. He saw how the design of the bones in the skull permitted slight motion, and how any restriction of normal motion due to injury, trauma, or disease could affect health. In the 1970s Dr John Upledger scientifically confirmed this theory and developed cranio-sacral therapy. This works to enhance the functioning of the central nervous system through releasing restrictions in the cranio-sacral system, comprised of the membranes and cerebrospinal fluid that surround and protect the brain and spinal cord. Some success has been reported with cranial sacral osteopathy in cases of glue ear, as it can release restrictions of the ossicles in the middle ear. It is usually recommended in combination with a low mucous forming diet.

Cysts: Fluid-filled sacs which may occur normally in tissues from time to time, or which may grow up around irritations in tissues. Sebaceous cysts (filled with sebum) are quite common harmless cysts, often found on the scalp.

Decibel: A unit of measure for the loudness of a sound, comparing the relative strength of two signals, or the relative strength of a signal compared to a standard signal value.

Desquamation: The shedding or peeling of the outer layer of the skin from the stratum corneum, as in exfoliation.

Dermatitis: The terms 'eczema' and 'dermatitis' are often used interchangeably. Atopic dermatitis, or eczema, is a chronic disease that causes areas of red, itchy skin. This condition usually starts in early childhood, especially when there is a family history of atopy (asthma, hay fever, conjunctivitis or food allergies). The skin fails to hold in moisture, becoming dry, inflamed, itchy and often infected. Hereditary dry skin and allergies leading to an overactive immune system are the most common causes.

Diabetes: A hereditary or developmental disease in which the body cannot convert food into energy because of a lack of insulin (a hormone produced by the pancreas), or because of an inability to use insulin. Diabetes is a serious condition that can cause complications ranging from numbness through to loss of vision and coma. It also significantly raises the risk for other problems, such as stroke and heart disease. Caution is advised in massaging due to the lack of sensation, particularly in hands and feet.

Juvenile diabetes, or type 1 diabetes, is treated with diet, exercise and insulin. Type 2, formerly called adult onset, is now seen in overweight children. It is treated with diet, exercise and medication. In severe cases, type 2 diabetes is also treated with insulin.

Diverticulitis: A condition in which pouch-like bulges or pockets (diverticula) in the wall of the intestine, most commonly the large intestine or colon, become infected or inflamed.

Eczema: See 'dermatitis'.

Electromagnetic energy: Electric and magnetic force field that surrounds a moving electric charge. Humans produce micro pulses of electrical charge with each movement, thought or emotion, and the basic rule of physics is that every electrical charge produces a corresponding electromagnetic field. The human electromagnetic field can be detected by Kirlian photography.

Endogenic: Derived or originating internally, as opposed to exogenic (externally). An exogenic stress factor would be environmental pollution, whereas an endogenic stress factor would be worry. Exogenic stress factors can lead to endogenic stress. Endogenic 'drugs' are substances produced naturally within the body such as endorphins, while the exogenic equivalent is morphine.

Endorphins: Natural substances, chemically similar to morphine, that the brain releases to relieve pain and bring about a feeling of wellbeing. The word literally means 'endogenous morphine' or morphine produced within the body. Touch therapies and exercise have been shown to raise endorphin levels in the body.

Eustachian tube: The tube (approximately. 3.5 cm long in adults, shorter in children) which connects the middle ear and the back of the nose, draining the middle ear and maintaining equal air pressure on both sides of the tympanic membrane (eardrum). If clogged by mucus, equalisation is hindered and there may be pain, deafness and sometimes a build-up of fluid in the middle ear (glue ear).

Fibromyalgia: A chronic disorder characterised by widespread musculoskeletal pain, fatigue, and multiple tender points that occur in precise, localised areas, particularly in the neck, spine, shoulders, and hips; also may cause sleep disturbances, morning stiffness, irritable bowel syndrome, anxiety, and other symptoms. Fibromyalgia affects females more than males.

Folliculitis: An inflammation of the hair follicles due to an infection or irritation. On the beard it is called folliculitis or sycosis barbae. Using a good shaving cream can help reduce this type of folliculitis.

Gall bladder: A pear-shaped muscular sac attached to and beneath the liver, which stores bile produced in the liver until needed by the body for digestion. Bile helps to break down fats in the digestive system.

Ginkgo biloba: The ginkgo is the oldest living tree species, and Chinese monks are credited with keeping the tree in existence as a sacred herb. It was first brought to Europe in the 1700s and is now a commonly prescribed drug in France and Germany. Following many studies, ginkgo is gaining recognition as a brain tonic that enhances memory because of its positive effects on the vascular system in the brain. It is also used as a treatment for vertigo, tinnitus (ringing in the ears) and a variety of neurological disorders and circulation problems. Ginkgo works by increasing blood flow to the brain (which uses 20 per cent of the body's oxygen) and throughout the body's network of blood vessels that supply blood and oxygen to the organ systems.

Gravity: The force that tends to draw all bodies in the earth's sphere toward the centre of the earth.

Grommets: A grommet is needed when the Eustachian tube is not working properly, leading to cases of 'glue ear' (a build-up of fluid in the middle ear). Grommets are tiny ventilation tubes which are inserted into the eardrum, allowing the fluid to drain out into the ear canal. This also allows air to pass freely into the middle ear, keeping the pressure at atmospheric levels and preventing deafness. The operation is usually done as a day case, under general anaesthetic.

Herpes simplex: Herpes simplex virus type 1 (HSV1) causes cold sores which are infections of the lips, mouth, and face. It is the most common herpes simplex virus and is usually acquired in childhood. It is transmitted by contact with infected saliva. By adulthood, up to 90 per cent of individuals will have antibodies to HSV-1.

Herpes simplex virus 2 (HSV-2) is sexually transmitted with symptoms including genital ulcers or sores. In addition to oral and genital lesions, the virus can also lead to complications such as meningoencephalitis (infection of the lining of the brain and the brain itself) or cause infection of the eye – in particular the conjunctiva and cornea. However, some people have HSV-2 but do not display symptoms.

Hippocrates: Hippocrates (c460–380 BC) was an Ancient Greek physician, regarded as one of the most outstanding figures in medicine of all time; he has been called 'the father of medicine.' He was a physician from the so-called medical school of Kos. In his writings, he rejected the superstition and magic of primitive 'medicine' and laid the foundations of medicine as a branch of science.

Homeopathic effect: In homeopathic medicine, there is a principle that 'like cures like', meaning that small, highly diluted quantities of medicinal substances are given to cure symptoms, when the same substances given at higher or more concentrated doses could actually cause those symptoms. The minute quantities of substances such as beeswax present in ear candles can have a beneficial effect on individuals who may be allergic to beeswax in large quantities. Hence, there are very few reported allergic reactions to ear candling.

Hormone: A chemical produced in one part of the body and released into the blood to trigger or regulate particular functions in another part of the body. For example, insulin is a hormone made in the pancreas that tells other cells when to use glucose for energy.

Hydrating: Restoring or maintaining the normal proportion of fluid.

Hypothalamus: A small structure at the base of the brain that regulates many body functions, including appetite and body temperature. Together with the pituitary gland, it also regulates the formation and release of many hormones in the body, including oestrogens and progesterone by the ovaries and testosterone by the testes.

Immune system: The body's system of defences against disease composed of certain organs, white blood cells and antibodies.

Antibodies are protein substances that react against bacteria and other harmful material.

Impetigo: A highly contagious bacterial skin infection characterised by small pus-filled blisters that form honey-yellow crusts. Using an antibacterial ointment can treat early impetigo.

Inferior vena cava: A large vein that carries de-oxygenated blood from the lower half of the body into the heart. The vein connects to the heart at a valve attached to the right atrium.

Initiation rites: Nearly every culture in the world ritualises the important milestones throughout life. Birth, marriage and death are typically marked by special ceremonies called initiation rites or rites of passage. The final passage from childhood to adulthood also figures prominently among various ethnic groups worldwide. The Hopi Indians and other cultures used ear candles in initiation rites.

Ions: Ions are atoms or molecules which carry an electrical charge. Positive ions attract atmospheric pollutants, dust particles and harmful airborne matter into interior spaces and keeps them there. Negative ions, which are abundant in natural places such as forests, waterfalls and the seaside, cancel the effect of positive ions and clean the air, increasing the sense of wellbeing. Ear candling is said to produce negative ions.

Labyrinth: The labyrinth is a system of fluid passages in the inner ear comprising the vestibular system and the auditory system, which provides the sense of balance. In Greek mythology, the labyrinth was an elaborate maze constructed for King Minos of Crete, and the labyrinth in the ear is so-called because of its maze-like appearance.

Laryngitis: Inflammation of the mucous membranes of the larynx (voice box) which may be accompanied by throat dryness, soreness, hoarseness, cough, and/or difficulty in swallowing.

Ligament: A band of fibrous tissue that connects bone to bone or cartilage to bone, supporting or strengthening a joint.

109

Lymph nodes: Small, bean-sized organs of the immune system, also called lymph glands, which are distributed widely throughout the body. Lymph fluid is filtered through the lymph nodes in which all types of lymphocytes take up temporary residence.

Lymphocytes: a type of white blood cell that plays a major role in the body's immune system. Includes B cells, which develop in the bone marrow and produce antibodies, and T cells, which develop in the thymus gland and are essential for the control and development of immune response.

Malaria: Malaria is a disease of the red blood cells caused by a parasite transmitted by the bite of an infected anopheles mosquito. These mosquitoes are present in the tropics and subtropics in almost all countries. Malaria is the most deadly of all tropical parasitic diseases. Symptoms include shivering, fever, sweating and anaemia as red blood cells are destroyed. There is currently no vaccine and preventative drugs include chloroquine and proguanil. Homeopathic remedies are also available.

Measles: A highly contagious viral disease characterised by fever, general weakness, sneezing, nasal congestion, a brassy cough, conjunctivitis, and a rash over the entire body. An attack of measles almost invariably confers permanent immunity to the disease. German measles, also known as rubella, is a contagious viral disease that is a milder form of measles. If contracted by a pregnant mother during the first trimester, it can cause permanent damage to the hair cells in the cochlea of the foetus, leading to deafness.

Meningitis: Inflammation of the membranes that cover the brain or spinal cord, usually caused by viral or bacterial infection.

Meridians: Acupressure and acupuncture, as well as other therapies such as shiatsu and reflexology, are based on the concept of a person's energy, or life force. This belief system theorises that a life force, known as chi or qi (pronounced chee) travels through the body along pathways called meridians. Traditional Chinese medicine dictates that there are 20 meridians. However, in acupressure and acupuncture, most work centres on 14 meridians. Eight of these meridians have points on the face.

Metastases: The spread of disease or tumour cells from one part of the body to another unrelated part of the body by the way of the bloodstream or lymphatic vessels.

Multiple sclerosis: A chronic, potentially debilitating disease in which the body's immune system attacks the protective coating (myelin) on nerve fibres within the central nervous system. It results in multiple scars, or scleroses, on the myelin sheath, leading to impairment or loss of nerve function.

Mumps: A viral infection that causes the salivary glands, especially the parotid gland, to swell. It is accompanied by fever, headache and vomiting and usually affects children. The infection may in some cases spread to other salivary glands, the pancreas and the testicles causing orchitis, which is inflammation of the testes.

Myringoplasty (or **tympanoplasty**): Surgical repair with a tissue graft of the eardrum.

Myringotomy: A minor surgical procedure in which a small slit is made in the eardrum, allowing fluid to drain from the middle ear; it may or may not involve placement of grommets (ventilating tubes).

Naturopathic: Naturopathic medicine proposes that there is a healing power in the body that establishes, maintains and restores health. Practitioners work with the patient to support this power, through treatments such as nutrition and lifestyle counselling, dietary supplements, medicinal plants, exercise, homeopathy, and treatments from traditional Chinese medicine. Some naturopathic practitioners are also qualified in orthodox medicine.

Neolithic: A period covering the years from about 3,200 BC to 1,800 BC. Neolithic literally means 'New Stone Age' and covers the time between the Mesolithic (Middle Stone Age) and the Bronze Age. In Europe the Neolithic age is characterised by the advent of farming. This led to a more settled way of life with permanent villages and the building of stone monuments such as stone circles and chambered tombs.

Olfactory: Relating to the sense of smell.

Oral thrush: Oral thrush is an infection of yeast fungus, candida albicans, in the mucous membranes of the mouth.

Ossiculoplasty: This is ear bone repair or replacement with an artificial substitute, which is used to repair the middle ear bones. Infection or damage to the tympanic membrane often damages the middle ear bones. In this case, the eardrum is repaired at the same time. Trauma may dislocate the ear bones without creating a hole in the eardrum. In this case, only the ear bones are repaired. Results of replacement of the incus and malleus are around 70 per cent. However, if the stapes is lost the success rate of the operation reported by some authors is under 50 per cent.

Otologist: A physician who is trained in otolaryngology (the study of the ear, nose, and throat) and who has specialised in problems relating to the ear.

Oxytocin: A hormone secreted by the pituitary gland that stimulates contractions of the uterus during childbirth and the milk-eject reflex. Pitocin is the synthetic form of this hormone, given to induce childbirth contractions.

Parasympathetic nervous system (PNS): One of two divisions of the autonomic nervous system, which operates without our conscious control. It conserves energy as it slows the heart rate, increases intestinal and gland activity, and relaxes sphincter muscles. It is stimulated by relaxation and touch therapies such as ear candling and massage, and acts to reverse the effects of the sympathetic nervous system, which has the opposite effects and is activated in times of stress.

Parkinson's disease: A progressive neurological condition affecting movements such as walking, talking and writing. It is named after Dr James Parkinson (1755–1824), the London doctor who first identified Parkinson's as a specific condition. Parkinson's has three main symptoms: tremor, which usually begins in one hand or arm; muscular rigidity or stiffness; and bradykinesia, meaning slowness of movement. People with Parkinson's may experience other symptoms such as tiredness, depression, difficulties with handwriting and other forms of communication such as speech, facial expression, and balance.

Pathogens: Organisms such as bacteria, viruses, parasites, or fungi that cause disease. Some bacteria pathogens are food-borne, such as salmonella.

Pediculosis capitis: Commonly known as head lice, these are tiny insects that live on the scalp. They can be spread by close contact with other people.

Peristalsis: The wavelike motion of muscles in the digestive tract, which moves the food along to be digested. In the stomach, this motion mixes food with gastric juices, turning it into a thin liquid called chyme.

Pineal gland: An endocrine organ found in the brain that secretes a hormone called melatonin, which is believed to control the biological rhythms (body clock) of the body. The pineal gland begins to shrink and calcify during the ageing process, thereby reducing the amount of circulating melatonin – probably one of the reasons we sleep less as we age.

Pituitary gland: A gland at the base of the brain that secretes hormones and regulates and controls other hormone-secreting glands and many body processes, including reproduction.

Pliny: (23–79 AD) Roman author of an encyclopaedia of natural history who died while observing the eruption of Mount Vesuvius in Sicily.

Precursor: a substance from which another usually more active or mature substance is formed. For example, the ultra-violet rays of the sun convert a precursor substance in the skin into Vitamin D.

Psoriasis: A chronic, non-contagious disease that occurs when the growth of new skin cells rapidly accelerates (from the average 28 days to just four days) resulting in thick, red, scaly, inflamed patches on the skin surface. It generally affects the extensor surfaces of the elbows, knees as well as the scalp, and around or in the ears, navel, genitals or buttocks. Approximately 10–15 per cent of patients with psoriasis develop joint inflammation (psoriatic arthritis). Psoriasis is thought to be an autoimmune condition. There is currently no cure, but many treatment options are available. As it is exacerbated by stress, touch therapies which relax are very comforting.

Reflex points: Points on the body that initiate an involuntary response to a stimulus such as touch or pressure. Reflexology is based on the principle that there are reflex points on the feet and hands that correspond and connect to all the organs, glands and parts of the body; and that by applying pressure to these points, the body is encouraged to heal naturally. The ear is rich in reflex points, and some therapists specialise in ear acupuncture or ear reflexology to promote healing.

Reiki: The word comes from two Japanese words – Rei and Ki, meaning universal life force energy. It is based on the principle that, by channelling spiritual energy through the practitioner, the spirit is healed, and the spirit in turn heals the physical body.

Residue: The dry solids remaining after evaporation or vaporisation. In the case of ear candles, the residue is beeswax and powder from the herbs infused in the candle.

Scabies: An intensely itching rash caused by a tiny mite (bug) that lives in the skin. Since it is only one-sixtieth of an inch long, the scabies mite is almost impossible to see without magnification. The rash usually involves the hands, wrists, breasts, genital area, and waistline. In severe cases scabies can spread to almost the entire body, but rarely affects the face. Scabies are spread through linens, clothes or close contact with infected people, and are treated with prescription lotions or soaps.

Scar tissue (adhesions): The body tissue remaining after a wound has healed. It is usually stronger than the original tissues, but less able to carry out the jobs that the original tissues were designed for.

Sebum: An oily secretion manufactured by tiny sebaceous glands near the hair follicles that lubricates and protects the hair and skin, preventing dryness and irritation.

Spleen: An organ which is part of the lymphatic system. The spleen produces lymphocytes to help fight infection and which filters the blood, stores blood cells and destroys old red blood cells. It is located on the left side of the abdomen near the stomach. It is not essential to life, but if removed may weaken the immune system.

Subtle energy: The vital energy or life force that permeates all living things including plants, animals, and humans.

Surrogate: A substitute or stand-in for the real thing. A surrogate mother carries a foetus that was conceived by another female and then implanted in her uterus.

Tai Chi: Tai Chi combines movement, meditation and breath regulation to enhance the flow of vital energy in the body, improve blood circulation, and enhance immune functions. It is estimated that 200 million Chinese people practice Tai Chi everyday.

Thrombosis: Formation of a blood clot (thrombus) in an artery or vein. The thrombus can obstruct the flow of blood in the vessel. Parts of the blood clot can also become detached from the clot and carried by the bloodstream to other sites (embolism). If a thrombus or embolus blocks a blood vessel supplying a vital organ, this can result in pulmonary embolism, heart attack or stroke depending on the site of the blockage.

Thymus: An organ that is part of the lymphatic system located in the chest behind the breastbone. Specialised white blood cells of the immune system called T lymphocytes grow and multiply here in infancy and childhood.

Tinea capitis: A fungal infection also known as ringworm of the scalp which usually manifests itself as a sharp and clearly defined patch of partial hair loss. The fungus invades the hair shaft and causes the hairs to break.

Inflammation and scaling may be present. The infection may be transmitted through combs, brushes, and from person to person.

Tonsillitis: An infection and subsequent inflammation of the tonsils, which are areas of lymphoid tissue on either side of the throat. Lymphoid tissue is part of the body's immune system, containing specialised white blood cells called lymphocytes that help to fight infection.

Trigeminal neuralgia: An extremely painful condition caused by a disturbance in the function of the trigeminal nerve (fifth cranial nerve) which carries sensation from your face to your brain. The pain is similar to an electric shock. Caution is advised when massaging the face.

Tuberculosis: An infection caused by bacteria called mycobacterium tuberculosis. Many people infected with tuberculosis have no symptoms because it is dormant. Once active, tuberculosis causes damage to the lungs and other organs. Active tuberculosis is also contagious and is spread through inhalation. Treatment of tuberculosis usually involves taking medication and vitamins for at least six months.

Vacuum: An enclosed space from which air has been removed; sound cannot travel through a vacuum so we know that ear candles do not create a vacuum in the ear canal because we can hear the sound of the ingredients vapourising.

Vapourised: Converted into a gas or vapour; the gaseous form of materials that are normally liquids or solids at room temperature and pressure.

Vasodilation: The widening or relaxing of blood vessels. This lowers blood pressure and eases the heart's workload. Massage encourages vasodilation of blood vessels in the skin.

Vascularisation: The stimulation of blood vessels within a body tissue.

Vertigo: A sense of spinning or dizziness, often accompanied by nausea and occasionally vomiting and is generally worsened by motion. It is sometimes caused by blood vessel compression of the vestibular nerve (nerve of balance).

Volatile: The term volatile is commonly understood to mean that a material evaporates easily, eg essential oils.

Whiplash: An injury to the ligaments, vertebrae or spinal cord in the neck region caused by sudden forward/backward jerking of the head and neck, often in occupants of a car hit from behind. Headrests can prevent this injury from happening. Clients with undiagnosed whiplash injuries should be referred to the doctor or hospital before treating.

Yoga: This name comes from the Sanskrit 'yeung', meaning unity or joining together. It is a Hindu philosophy used to attain spiritual insight and harmony, but in common use it refers to a system of exercises practised as part of this discipline.

index

Page numbers in italics refer to pictures and diagrams.

Enjoyed this? Then visit our website for information on our other *In Essence* titles

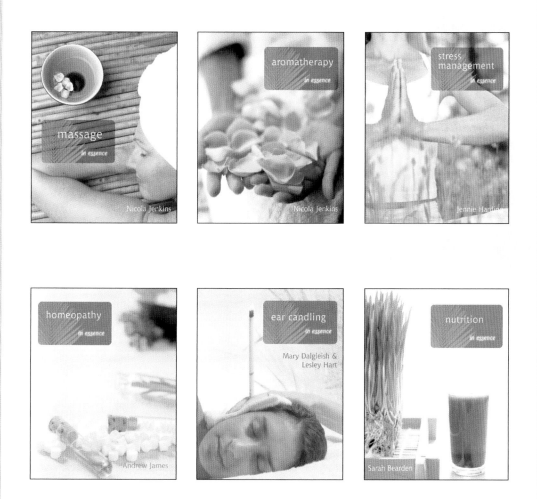

Indulge yourself
www.hoddereducation.co.uk/FE/Therapies

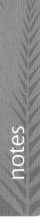
notes